Tricks... To Please a Man

by Jay Wiseman

greenery press

Cover, Johnny Ink Design, www.johnnyink.com.

Published in the United States by Greenery Press, 3403 Piedmont Ave. #301, Oakland, CA 94611, www.greenerypress.com.

ISBN 1-890159-52-2

contents

Acknowledgments

This book is dedicated to Baraka Jaden, who has always lovingly been there for me, particularly in time of great need, and who helps keep me honest (and who is an excellent Trickster). Here's to our past, our present, and our future.

All of the people listed below also helped to a significant degree in one way or another, and sometimes in more than one way, in helping this book to become a reality. Some contributed material, some contributed much-needed support (including baby-sitting the author when necessary), some acted as sounding boards and reality checkers, some did part of the above, and some did all of the above. My grateful thanks to you all.

Andrew Conway
Atheris
Baraka Jaden
Bill Burns
Bert Herrman (who inspired this version)
Cecilia Tan
Charles Moser, Ph.D., M.D.
Deborah Addington
Don't Tell Them Where You Got That
Francesca Guido
Glenna
Gretchen Rau

Janet Hardy
Joanne
John and Libby Warren
Karen Mendelsohn
Kathy Labriola
Keep My Name Out Of It
Lady Elle from St. Louis
Lady Sarah
Linda K.
Lynn Craig
Maggi Rubenstein, Ph.D.
Margaret aka KitNBoots
Mic and Beth

Mike Peterman
Mistress Lorelei
Nightlace
Oberon & Morning Glory Zell
Rachael Brennan
Robin Stewart
Sage
Silk of Dallas

Susannah C. of Hartford (I promised you that I'd remember you, and I always and fondly will)
Tammy Jo Eckhart
Tom & Katy Burns
Walter Shelbourne
Wendy H. of Marin

Warning and Disclaimer

There is no such thing as risk-free sex, especially these days. Sexual behavior, and the personal, interpersonal, and broader implications of what it means, can be intense, powerful matters.

In the medical world, there's a dictum about administering medication that involves "the five rights": Give the right drug to the right patient at the right time in the right dosage by the right method. A similar outlook can apply to sexual behavior. Being sexual with the right person, in the right way, at the right time, in the right location, and for the right reasons can be an incredibly positive experience for everyone involved. If any of the above is not right, however, then problems – sometimes very severe or even life-destroying problems – can emerge.

Erotic energy is one of the most powerful forces in our world. Respect and pay attention to that power and you can experience bliss. Disrespect or ignore that power and you might not live to regret it.

The primary purpose of "Tricks to Please A Man" is to provide information and advice that will help make good sex between informed, consenting adults a little bit better. It also provides basic information to help people understand their situations, make them aware of possible alternatives, cope with problems, and find helpful resources.

Please do not think of this book as any kind of medical, legal, psychological, or other professional advice. It most certainly is not intended as a substitute for proper sex therapy. Most of its core information, particularly the "tricks" themselves, was discovered by me, taught to me by lovers, shared with me by friends during highly informal conversations (many has been the time since the first "Tricks" book was published that someone has come up to me and said "I've got a trick for you"), or sent to me either in the mail or over the Internet. Please keep that in mind when considering this book's contents.

Almost without question, there are at least a few factual errors in this book, and probably some typographical errors as well. Also, it's very common, in this and many other fields, that information believed to be accurate at the time of publication is later revealed to be inaccurate – sometimes only slightly so, sometimes very much so. If you have even the slightest doubt about the accuracy or safety of anything in this book, please check with independent sources. If their recommendations differ from mine, please let me know. By the way, please remember that not all professional advice is equally complete, accurate, up-to-date, and unbiased. By all means get an independent "second opinion" (and maybe even a "third opinion") if you feel even the slightest need for it.

No one associated with writing, editing, printing, distributing, or selling this book is in any way liable for any damages that result from you acting on the information herein. While I have most certainly not put anything in here that I consider likely to be harmful, *understand clearly that the information herein is presented "as is" and "with all faults"* and that you act on the information in this book entirely at your own risk.

Feedback please!

If you think you have found a factual error, typographical error, or other inaccuracy or omission in this book, please let me know so that this can be corrected in future printings.

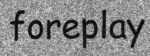foreplay

introduction: 750 tricks later...

It's been a bit more than eleven years since the first Tricks book was published. It was a fun book – fun to research, fun to write, fun to publish, and fun to market. Yet it was also important. Feedback revealed that the book helped people to have fun, and also helped people to be a little more mindful of how they participated in sex. That was a good thing.

At the time, of course, I thought the book would be a one-shot kind of thing. I don't see how I could have anticipated that the book would lead to the subsequent writing and publishing of "Tricks 2," and then "Sex Toy Tricks," and then "Supermarket Tricks." All of those books helped thousands of people in many different ways. I'm happy and I'm proud of them.

With the publication of "Tricks... to Please a Man" as a companion volume for "Tricks... to Please a Woman," we have now entered a sort of era of the next generation of Tricks books. Will there be more? I honestly don't know. The general framework and paradigm of the first Tricks book seems to have inspired a number of other authors, but somehow the Tricks books still stand on their own, with the very special voice with which they speak perhaps imitated but never surpassed.

So here I sit, the author of a six-volume set of books on sex tricks. There are days when I wonder how in the world *that* happened. While every step in that journey made sense at the time I took it – and, in retrospect, still does – the journey has led me to a very interesting and unique place.

So, what has the journey taught me?

First, it has taught me that our sexuality comes from a very deep place within our beings. I wonder if anything else, except possibly for our religious and spiritual beliefs, comes from a deeper place. Our sexuality addresses some of the very core issues of who we are as people.

Second, the sexual energy that comes from this very deep place within us is very powerful and must be treated with the respect owed to that power. This is a very strong, vital force. Perhaps it must be so to accomplish the goals of a happy and satisfying sex life.

Third, to treat this energy with the respect it deserves, we must address it mindfully. This is something it is wise to think about, and to reflect upon at length. We must address it both intellectually and emotionally, and doing that necessarily involves making ourselves vulnerable. Doing so pays off. I have had the opportunity to talk with a very large number of people about their sexuality, and I have noticed a distinct correlation between how in touch with and comfortable about their sexuality they were, and their overall level of mindfulness and cluefulness.

Fourth, sexuality is much more than a series of tricks that have been strung together. Think of tricks as the sprinkles that are on top of the icing that is on top of the cake. While it's fun to enjoy the sprinkles, and also to enjoy the icing, don't confuse them with the deeper rewards of enjoying the cake.

My best wishes in your explorations. May all of your tricks make both you and your partner happier.

Jay Wiseman
San Francisco, California
September, 2003

about tricks

Creativity expert Edward DeBono once pointed out that a good way to improve a situation was to look at some aspect of it that was already working well and to figure out how to make it work even better (thus disproving the self-defeating cliche, "If it's not broken, don't fix it").

Back in 1992, I decided to apply that concept to sex. It only took me a moment to realize that virtually every lover of mine had something she did to improve our sex life just slightly. It might have been a special way that she used her hand or her mouth, or a particular way she arranged things, or how she smoothed out something that would otherwise have been awkward. I also saw that, over the years, I had thought of several on my own. I named these behaviors "tricks" and decided to write a book about them.

Thus, in October of 1992, the book was born. I named it "Tricks: More Than 125 Ways to Make Good Sex Better." It was a delightful little book, fun to write (and to research!), easy to market, and just generally pleasant all the way around. What I didn't suspect at the time was that I had created an ever-so-gentle monster – a monster that gradually began to take on a life of its own.

My friends started coming up to me and saying "I've got a trick for you." Occasionally, during our own lovemaking, my partner or I would say "hey, that's a trick." (I kept a notepad by our bed.) People sent me tricks in the mail. Eventually, the situation reached "critical mass" and over the next three years, I published three more books in the series: "Tricks 2," "Sex Toy Tricks" and "Supermarket Tricks."

Many years later, I decided to revisit those books. I decided that the information in them would be more useful if it were organized by the gender of the recipient, and that furthermore, I'd heard a lot of great ideas in the intervening years. Hence: "Tricks... To Please a Woman," and this companion volume, "Tricks... To Please A Man." These books were both written primarily for the heterosexual reader, although I hope that gay men, lesbians and bisexuals will find many of their contents helpful.

This book contains 125 tricks, plus as many suggestions, resources and nuggets of information as we could cram between the covers. Relatively few of them, at this point, originated with me – they've been submitted by women and men of various sexual orientations and backgrounds.

It's not impossible that there will be sequels, so feel free to send in more tricks! You can write to me care of my publisher, Greenery Press – look at the copyright page or the last page of this book for contact information.

The Limits Of Tricks

You know, and I know, that lovemaking cannot be and should not be reduced to tricks. Tricks are to erotic play what spices are to eating: a few carefully chosen ones make the experience more intense and pleasurable, but too many can be overwhelming.

It's entirely possible to have a wonderful and completely satisfying sex life without knowing any of the tricks in this book, or any others.

Good sex is based on caring about your partner's well-being, really wanting to have sex with them (and, of course, your partner really wanting to have sex with you), and observing the responsibilities that go with that caring. Still, adding a carefully chosen spice now and then can make the sex even more fun.

Your underlying feelings towards the other person, and theirs toward you, greatly affect whether or not a trick will improve your erotic play. As one lady told me, "If I really like him, then he almost can't do anything wrong. If I really don't like him, then he can't even breathe right."

Tricks don't work well in isolation. Each person has their own erotic response pattern, something I've come to think of as their "envelope." One of your main tasks as a good lover is to find your partner's envelope. Something that is wildly erotic for one person can be grossly unpleasant for another.

The envelope varies widely from person to person. It also varies over time with the same person. An experience once thought repulsive can become highly attractive, and vice versa. Find their envelope before you try too many tricks, and remember that the location and content of that envelope change over time.

A Few Don'ts Regarding Tricks (and Other Matters)

•   Don't spend too much time doing tricks. It's far more important to stay in the here and now with your lover. Do a trick every now and then, as the occasion arises.

•   Don't try to do too many different tricks in a single session. Again, doing so can distance you from your lover.

• Don't be overly concerned with looking for opportunities to do a trick. Let such opportunities appear naturally during the course of lovemaking. Men seem particularly vulnerable to this pitfall – thus giving rise to the somewhat bitter saying among many women, "There were three of us in bed: me, him, and his technique."

• Never place anything in a woman's vagina if it's recently been in her (or, for that matter, any other person's) rectum. Doing so can cause an infection that will require a visit to a doctor and antibiotics to cure. For example, using your penis, fingers or sex toy on her anus and then her vagina would be very likely to cause such an infection. Anything used for anal play must first be thoroughly cleaned before it can be used for vaginal play. (See the "Afterplay" section for more information on toy cleaning.)

• Never seal your mouth over a woman's vagina and blow air into it. There are reports of women suffering fatal air embolisms from this practice. Menstruating and pregnant women seem to face a considerably higher than average risk. Such incidents are very, very rare, but they do happen.

• Be careful about placing food items in a woman's vagina, especially sugary foods. Many men and women recommended placing various foods in there and then eating them out. (Grapes have something of a cult following.) These foods can upset the natural balance and cause infections, particularly yeast infections. You can do such tricks if you want, but if you do, then understand that you may have to deal with their effects "the morning after."

• *Use intoxicants judiciously if at all.* Light intoxicant use can relax you, brighten your mood, and help release your inhibitions. More-than-light intoxicant use is asking for trouble: your judgment becomes dangerously cloudy, your coordination suffers, your nerve endings are dulled... you may become too out of it to be sexual at all. Even worse, intoxication can impair your judgment about sexual risk-taking, leading you to have unsafe sex that you wouldn't consider while sober. And remember – having sex with someone too drunk or stoned to understand what's happening just might get you charged with rape.

assumptions

In presenting the information in this book, I am making the following assumptions about your situation. If these assumptions are not true in your case, please adjust your behavior accordingly. I'm assuming:

• That both of you are willing (and, hopefully, eager) to have sex with each other. Consent is absolutely essential.

• That having sex with each other will not violate any agreements you have made with other people about your sexual conduct.

• That both of you understand the nature of what you are doing. Having sex with someone too young, mentally impaired, senile, intoxicated, or otherwise unable to understand and consent to what is happening may get you charged with rape, even if no force was used. Remember, if he (or she) is too drunk to drive, he may be too drunk to have sex.

• That both of you have reached the age of consent in your state (and that you live in the United States). I believe the age of consent is as low as 14 in at least one state and as high as 18 in many others. Remember, an act that is perfectly legal on one side of a state line might get you a lengthy prison sentence on the other side. Make certain you know the age of consent in your state.

• That the acts I'm describing are legal in your state. Although the laws are rarely enforced, oral sex, anal intercourse and other practices are still a crime in some states, even if done by consenting adults in private. Find out your state's laws (and, where appropriate, work to change them). Your local library should have a copy of your state's criminal code in its reference section; you may also be able to find this information on the Internet (try *www.findlaw.com* to get started). Reading its sections on rape, incest, indecent exposure, lewd and lascivious conduct, assault, contributing to the delinquency of a minor, and related sections may be very informative. Asking a local attorney or police officer can also help, but remember that opinions, knowledge, and objectivity can vary widely, even among such "experts." Try to talk to more than one source.

• That there is no risk of passing on a sexually transmitted disease. If such a risk does exist, please modify what you do. Among other things, if you have herpes or have tested positive for the AIDS virus and have sex with someone without first telling them about that, you could be arrested. You could also face a lawsuit if your partner becomes infected. If you have any questions, one resource is the National Sexually Transmitted Disease and AIDS Hotline at (800) 227-8922.

fade in

Imagine that you are at an informal dinner party for ten highly open-minded people. You know five of the other people there, but not the other four. None of you is a health-care professional.

The food (quite delicious, by the way) has been served and the guests are now lingering over the remnants of their desserts, coffee, and after-dinner drinks. The conversation, somehow or other, turns to sex play. One of the husbands describes something he does that drives his wife (who is sitting next to him) crazy in bed. She blushes a bit, but is not really angry. Instead, she pipes up with, "Oh, yeah? Well let me tell you what turns him on." She then proceeds to do exactly that, and it's now his turn to blush a little.

This exchange, as such exchanges often do, prompts another guest to share one of their favorite bedroom pleasures, and now the whole table joins in with enthusiasm.

Dozens of comments follow, incorporating such phrases as "I just love it when someone…" and "I know I can always drive a guy wild when I…" Other comments include, "I just hate it when someone…" and "One thing I learned the hard way was…" And so it continues, for well over an hour. People pour out their special caresses, tricks they do with their mouths, ways to keep out of trouble, and special techniques for adding extra heat to an already hot situation.

When the conversation finally lapses, there's a moment of slightly embarrassed silence, and the dinner party begins to break up. A few of the couples, their eyes slightly smoldering, seem in a politely eager hurry to return to their homes. One of the men makes a few discreet notes on a napkin. At this point, the scene fades out.

I want you to regard the tricks and other information in this book much as you would regard what you would hear at such a dinner party. None of it is any sort of professional or expert advice, but most of it seems to make sense – and of course you will independently check on matters you have questions about before trying them yourself.

14 foreplay

basic tricks

"Two warm bodies in a bed" – what could be more basic, or more wonderful, than that? This section includes a few fine points of male anatomy and psychology that may be unfamiliar to my female readers, as well as a few ideas for using parts of your bodies that otherwise might not get quite enough use in the boudoir.

1 Use Your Words

Many male Tricksters, and more than a few female ones, note that men really appreciate it when women don't expect their guys to be mind-readers. Ladies, don't just lie back and wait for him to figure out what feels good to you; be verbal, and specific, about what you want. If it's too hard, say so. Too soft, say so. Need more speed or less, say so. This is an acquired skill, and may seem a bit awkward at first – but there's a way to do it so that it doesn't feel like you're barking orders. Tell him when what he's doing feels good, then tell him what he could do to make it feel even better: "Oooh, that's nice; try it a little harder… aah, yes, that's great!"

Don't Just Lie Back, Feedback!

Many men feel, and it's sadly sometimes true, that their sexual touch is not really wanted by the woman involved. They feel it is often something she is tolerating, perhaps with the thought of getting something in return. Therefore, a woman can do much to put a man at ease by reassuring him that she does indeed welcome his touch – assuming, of course, that this is indeed the case. (If it's not, they need to talk – probably outside the bedroom, and perhaps with the help of a counselor.) If she does genuinely want him, she can often use words very creatively. Many men love hearing encouraging phrases such as "harder," "deeper," and "take me!"

Baby Steps

If your man is like many others, he's been raised to believe it's "unmanly" to let anyone else take the lead in bed, or to accept any kind of attention to his body. If you start to be more assertive, he may indeed like it but feel confused. Go slowly, mark what he likes and mark what he doesn't. Always make sure he knows that what you are doing to him or for him turns you on.

Up, Down, Up, and Off

When setting up your bedroom to create "your own little world," it can help to run down the following checklist:

Turn *up* the heat. Many people need a temperature of at least 75 degrees to feel comfortable while naked.

Turn *down* the lights. Candles and low wattage bulbs are nice. Dimmer switches on regular lights can be useful. Drapes and blinds can be adjusted. Softer lights make the situation more intimate. Also, most of us look better under soft lighting than we look under a glaring spotlight.

Turn *up* the music. Again, this adds atmosphere. It also helps keep "unique" sounds private.

Turn *off* the phone's ringer. There is something about a ringing telephone that can be almost irresistible. Let your voice mail or answering machine take the call (and turn down the answering machine's volume).

Feeling Good All Over

For many men, the only touching that feels erotic to them is touching on their genitals. (For some men, it's only their penis. Even touching their scrotum doesn't feel erotic.) One good way to eroticize more of a man's body is to touch and stroke (or, perhaps, lick and suck) his penis and, as the same time, touch and stroke another part of his body. His scrotum, nipples, and inner thighs are good places to start. In many cases, pleasurable sensations will be built up over time.

One tip: Don't try to eroticize too many different places at the same time. Spend a few sessions on just his nipples, for example, before working on other areas.

Speak Up

Good sex is closely related to a person's ability to stay "here and now and involved in what's happening." Anything that interferes with that detracts from the experience. Correct anything that distracts or bothers you early, and as diplomatically as possible. Are you cold? Is the music too loud? Is your position uncomfortable? Correct those things before they grow from minor annoyances into serious disruptions.

Men's Chests Need Love Too

Several women reported to me that their men's chests, especially their nipples, were more sensitive to stroking, light scratching, licking, sucking, and friendly biting than the men thought.

Safewords

Safewords are special words lovers use to indicate that "the game" needs to be slowed down or stopped. They first became widespread in kinky circles, but are useful for all adventurous lovers.

To prevent possibly disastrous misunderstandings, lovers need special signals to indicate that one of them "really" needs to have what's going on slowed down or stopped. Safewords fill that need. Safewords are usually chosen from words not likely to otherwise come up. "Yellow" is often used to signal "let's ease up or slow down." "Red" is often used to signal "Stop what's going on. I *really* mean it." Failure to honor a safeword is an extremely serious matter – in some cases, it can even be a crime. *Never* joke or kid around with safewords.

9 Honey, I'm Moaning Now, Can You Tell?

A wise Trickster notes, "Men, of course, like to think that their partners are having a good time, but they sometimes have a hard time picking up on subtle signs of enjoyment. If you're enjoying yourself, let it show – don't overact, but don't hold back on noises, motions and other signs of pleasure. It will enhance his experience, and you may find it will enhance yours too."

10 A Warm, Wet Touch

Our genitals remain very sensitive after we've had sex. One thing that can feel wonderful is to moisten a washcloth with warm water and place it there. I once had a lover who, as I was lying there feeling somewhat exhausted, would get up, prepare the washcloth, and place it on me. Oh, bliss! To this day, I have fond memories of her.

Safety note: Make sure the water is comfortably warm, but not too hot! Test it on your own elbow before placing it on him.

11

Coming In/ Going Out

If you have sex just before you go out to a special evening event, you may have a special glow for the rest of the night.

12

Nipple Uses

Caress his cock and balls with one of your nipples. Or try caressing his nipples with one of yours.

13

Tubby Time

Set aside one evening to meet him at the door, undress him and lead him into the bathroom. Then put him in a prepared bathtub and give him a bath. Don't worry about being sexy, don't worry about money, don't talk about the kids. Just talk about his body, the feel of it, how the water and soap feels to you, get him out of his head and into his body with your touch and your words.

Depending on your guy and your relationship, you may want to let him know ahead of time, or surprise him. You decide.

14 Forty Lashes

Flutter your eyelashes against his various tender bits. Of course, the use of false eyelashes offers a very wide range of possibilities.

15 Before and After

During his orgasm, and for a few minutes afterward, the head of a man's penis is likely to be much more sensitive to touch than it is at other times. Therefore, any touching there is felt much more intensely than it is felt at other times – so much so that touching it may be painful. Some men like to have the head of their cock rubbed briskly when they come, some like to have it left alone, and some like to have it lightly stroked. Your partner can tell you which he likes. Just remember that strokes which felt wonderful to him before he reached orgasm may feel agonizing during and immediately afterward.

It's Story Time

Human beings love stories; it's one of the things that separate us from animals. During sex or foreplay – or at other times, like when you can't be together but are talking on the phone – use your mind and your voice to create pictures and people in his mind. Men, we are told, are very visual, and that's true – but you can use your imagination and your voice to create pictures inside his mind. Use his own fantasies and interests but tweak them to reflect what you like too; that way you not only tell him what he wants to hear but also give him something he can share with you later, if he's inspired to talk.

Advanced version: You start a story, perhaps based on a fantasy you know he likes, and get the action started… then, when things are going along nicely, pause, and let him do the next part. The two of you can take turns storytelling while you keep each other busy with your hands, mouths and other body parts. This game can be strung along for some time and can be creatively as well as sexually quite exciting.

Enter By The Side Or Rear

Seldom-touched parts of the body are often very soft and tender – and that very tenderness means that they often react erotically to gentle touch from fingers, tongues and toys. In keeping with this theory, let me report that the sides and rear wall of the scrotum are often wonderfully sensitive to light stroking by fingers or tongue.

Get Happy, Not Pregnant

If you're worried about the possibility of pregnancy, keep in mind that he may not want to have vaginal intercourse with you so much as he wants to have an orgasm – with your help. Skillful use of your hand and/ or mouth can often resolve the situation. (I can tell you that, in my own case, many is the time I would have happily accepted that solution.)

19 Hooker's Trick #1

One professional I interviewed told me that both she and her clients enjoy it when she undresses them. The usual pattern, she pointed out, is for the man to undress the woman and then to undress himself. Many men have never been undressed by a woman. They therefore find the experience, particularly if her eagerness makes her a bit "rough" while she does it, exciting and intense.

20 I Got Rhythm

One playful lady Trickster told me that her lovers really enjoy it if, during intercourse, she keeps time to the music by squeezing her vaginal muscles.

21 Manual Dexterity

If you have a hand free during intercourse, try enhancing the experience by using that hand to play with his balls or to penetrate his anus with a well-lubed finger.

22 Orgasm vs. Ejaculation

For many men, orgasm and ejaculation only overlap to a certain degree. (There are whole books and workshops about how to separate them entirely.)

In my case, for example, I have noticed that I sometimes ejaculate quite a bit at the very beginning of my orgasm, long before the feelings reach their peak. (Therefore, I probably shouldn't try to use the withdrawal method of birth control, nor should I promise to not come in my lover's mouth.) Furthermore, my orgasm lasts for nearly a minute, continuing for quite some time after I have stopped ejaculating. I once got slightly irked with a lover when she stopped masturbating me because "all the sperm had stopped coming out." I explained my situation to her, and we never had that problem again.

Remember, orgasm and ejaculation can be two separate things.

23 The Tip of the Iceberg

The penis offers more than meets the eye. The shaft extends farther back into the body; finding and stimulating the invisible parts of the shaft can provide an unaccustomed, surprising, pleasant sensation. Place your fingers behind the scrotum, and press up. You'll be able to feel the part of the shaft you can't see. Once you've got it between your fingers, slide back and forth. Lengthen your stroke to include the perineum, another neglected portion of the male anatomy (the perineum is the section of tissue between the scrotum and the anus and it's loaded with nerve endings). This particular stroke hits nerves from near the prostate gland and carries sensation all the way down to the tip of the penis. You may need lube for the longer stroke, so have some handy.

24 Slow and Spready

Many men have difficulty reaching orgasm if their legs are spread apart. If you're feeling mischievous, "make him earn it" by having him keep his legs spread wide while you use your hands and mouth.

25 There's A Point To All This

The spot on the underside of the penis, just below the notch in the head, is often exceptionally receptive to being licked and stroked. Tantra practitioners sometimes refer to this location as Osho's point, and make good use of it.

26 Ladies First

Given that many men "run out of steam" after they've had an orgasm, if he wants you to give him one through masturbation or fellatio, affectionately try the "ladies first" approach.

No, Thank You

Ladies, we all have our limits, and we all sometimes have to express them. But if you have to say "no" to a proposition of his, it's both kind and courteous to phrase your refusal in such a way that it's clear that the issue is yours, not his. Acting disgusted or shocked, or making fun of him, is often a surefire way to shut down any chance of sexual innovation between the two of you in the future.

Couch the refusal so as to make it clear that the lack is in you rather than him – and, perhaps, suggest an alternative that might be nearly as much fun and that *is* within your limits.

Red Light, Green Light

I still remember with delight a certain lady, many years ago – a Trickster before her time, I guess – who played a game with me where she told me, "I'll keep on doing this to you [and, no, I'm not going to tell you what "this" was; you can use your imagination] unless you move, but if you move even a tiny bit, I'll stop." It was one of the most excruciating, ecstatic experiences of my young life.

32 tricks

manual tricks

Our first, and often our best, sex toy is the one at the end of our arm. Masturbating our partners is almost completely safe, tremendously intimate, and intensely pleasurable – and the boundless creativity and enthusiasm of the many, many tricks I received in this area proved that a skillfully administered "hand job" is one of the great and timeless erotic arts.

29 Upsy Daisy

A very simple but effective trick: when masturbating a man, give his penis a slight squeeze on the upstroke, focusing on the circle made by your thumb and forefinger as they pass over the corona (the "crown" where the head and the shaft of the penis meet).

Pin The Skin

Grasp his erect penis with your thumb and forefinger just below its tip. (If you are right-handed, this would probably work best if you used your left hand.) Keep your grasp slightly firm, and slide your hand all the way down the shaft of his penis to its base. You should now have his penis in your hand with its skin pulled somewhat tight over it. You may see its head slightly but noticeably bulge when you pull the skin down.

Normally, when a man masturbates, gets his cock sucked, or has intercourse, this skin slides at least somewhat. Pinning the skin in place and then stimulating his penis produces a noticeably more intense, usually highly pleasurable, sensation. One caution: such stimulation may feel rough and unpleasant if his penis is dry, so use enough lubricant to keep things slippery, especially during masturbation.

Warm Hands, Warm Heart

Place your (unlubricated) hands palm to palm together in front of you so your fingers are pointing away from you, then rub them vigorously together in a front-to-back motion. The friction thus created warms your hands – some believe that it also generates erotic energy – and can thus make receiving your touch extra pleasurable. To further build this pleasure, rub them together for a full minute.

Thumb Strum

Sit between his legs and grasp his cock firmly in both hands, with your fingers between his cock and his stomach and your thumbnails facing toward the ceiling. Run the ball of each thumb in turn up the underside of his penis, from the root toward the head, lifting the thumb away from the penis when it reaches the head. This masturbation stroke gives him very intense stimulation to the sensitive underside of the head of his penis.

33 Up Close and Personal

Many couples especially like the position in which he lies on his back while she sits between his legs, his thighs draped over hers and his genitals very close to her tummy. The benefit here is that from this position her hands can reach a great deal of his skin.

34 A Movable Fist

This trick is useful when masturbating or performing oral sex on him. Make one hand into a fist and place it just behind his scrotum. The thumb side should point forward and the little finger side should point to his rear. Thrust upwards against his body. The strength of this thrust can be anywhere from very light to very heavy, depending on what works for both of you. The strength can also be varied. As an extra touch, you can vibrate your fist.

Ball Pull

While using your hand and/or mouth to pleasure his penis, encircle the top of his scrotum with the thumb and forefinger of your other hand. Squeeze this ring together until it's snug and his testicles are "trapped" below it. Slowly and lightly pull down until the skin of his scrotum is pulled tight over his testicles. Lightly pull just a little more for about five seconds while you continue to pleasure his penis, then release the pull (but keep your hand in place). Closely watch his face, breathing, and body for a reaction. Repeat, varying the strength and length of the pull while you mix it with large amounts of pleasure.

Men will vary considerably in their reaction to this Trick. Some will find it so painful as to be a turn-off and want you to stop. Others will like it and want you to continue. Some will *really* like it and want you to pull down harder. (Don't get carried away. This Trick, carried to an extreme, could damage him.) Getting feedback from him on how long and how hard he wants the pull to be is an excellent idea.

TesTickles

Once you have his balls "trapped" as described in the preceding Trick, you can lick, caress, and lightly scratch the tightly stretched skin over them to excellent effect.

Thumb Fun

Encircle the penis just below its head with your thumb and forefinger, with your thumb on the back of his penis. Rotate your index finger up and over the head of his penis and then back to where you started, keeping your thumb stationary.

This can be an intense, highly pleasurable trick.

38 Do The Twist

The lower edge of the head of a man's penis (the corona) is very sensitive to touch, perhaps the most sensitive part of all. Tongues, fingers, and other items can be used to good effect here.

One excellent way to make masturbation more intense and pleasurable is to give your hand a light twist as it passes over the corona in the down-to-up direction. To illustrate, make your hand into a loose fist with your thumb on top of your index finger. Hold this in front of you so that your thumb is pointed straight ahead. Now move your arm forward while you turn your fist so it's facing palm-up and slide your thumb slightly toward the floor. You have just done the basic twist. Use this twist lightly (too much pressure may spoil it) and you may dramatically improve the quality of the hand jobs you give. It is a very simple yet exceptionally powerful technique.

Back, *Then* Forth

One dextrous Trickster writes: "Another nice handjob trick is to change the normal up-and-down motion. Instead of rubbing down the length of the cock and then changing direction, use both hands alternately to rub in a downward direction for a while, so he'll feel like he's just going deeper and deeper and deeper, and then switch directions. (You really need lube for this.) I don't know if it works just because it feels good, or because it makes him feel like his cock is about a yard long."

Give Him A Wring

Grip his cock between your two (preferably well-lubricated) hands like you would grab a baseball bat. Your uppermost hand should include the top of his penis in your grip. Twist your hands together until your thumbs are almost touching, then twist your hands apart in a wringing motion until your thumbs are pointing in parallel-but-opposite directions. Repeat this stroke, varying speed and grip strength as appropriate.

41
Flat Top

Hold the shaft of his penis in one hand so that it points straight away from his body. Stiffen the palm and fingers of your other (well lubricated) hand and place your palm on the head of his penis. Lightly but firmly rub your palm to and fro, side to side, in clockwise circles, and in counter-clockwise circles. You can also tilt your hand front and rear or side to side.

This technique involves a lot of stimulation directly on one of the most sensitive parts of a man's body, so make sure it doesn't get so intense that it becomes unpleasant. Watching his face will give you clues.

42
Forearmed Is Foreplay

Hold his cock in one hand and rub it with the inside of your other arm's forearm. The extra smooth sensation can feel wonderful. (This may also work on his nipples.)

Make A Snake

Straighten out your hands as you might do while praying and hold his penis in between them. Then rub your hands back and forth, as you might do when handling cooking dough or modeling clay.

This Trick has great variability. You can change – among other things – how fast you rub your hands, when you start and stop, whether or not to include the sensitive head of his penis, and both what type and how much (if any) lubricant you use while doing this.

If you're feeling like being extra nice to him, take the head of his penis in your mouth while you apply this stroke to its shaft.

Milking It For All It's Worth

When a man has an orgasm, the sensations of his orgasm mix with the sensations of semen passing through his penis. Interestingly enough, his orgasm often doesn't pump all of his semen out of his penis: some remains behind.

During masturbation or fellatio, you can often give him a tiny "extra" orgasm by pinching his cock lightly but firmly and "milking" this remaining fluid from his penis after his "regular" orgasm has finished. You can even put your thumb on the base of his penis and your finger at the rear top of his scrotum and milk that section forward, then bring your hand forward and milk the penis from base to tip, producing a more complete emptying. (Be sure you don't painfully squeeze his testicles.) Your lover can try this when he masturbates to find what method feels best, then teach it to you.

This can also be done by him, and perhaps by you, after he has climaxed during vaginal or anal intercourse. Withdraw the penis most (not all) of the way, milk it, then reinsert. Ah, bliss.

45 Moo!

Many farm girls will know that milking is a wonderful technique to use on a cock. Grasp the cock with your whole hand, but instead of wrapping your thumb around, turn it downward, running parallel to the cock and pressing into it (so the tip of your thumb is near the head of the cock). Instead of moving your hand up and down the cock, stimulate it by pressing your fingers in a wave pattern. Very nice.

46 Olive Your Best

Olive oil can make a great lubricant for use in conjunction with masturbation (or, for that matter, fellatio). It's cheap. It tastes good. It maintains a good slickness. It's fun to compare and contrast the benefits of virgin olive oil and extra virgin olive oil. However, like all oils, it's not latex-friendly, so save it for use when there's no latex nearby.

Up and Down

47

This trick requires a bit of coordination at first, but is very powerful once you master it. If you watch a man masturbate, you'll see that he typically uses one hand to stroke his penis in an up and down motion. All well and good. You can add some variety and spice to this by using one of your hands only for upstrokes and the other only for downstrokes. Try this: have him lie on his back while you sit or kneel (whatever is comfortable) between his legs. Lubricate his penis and your hand well, then lightly grasp the base of his penis with your right hand and gently hold its tip with your left. Stroke upwards with your right hand. When your right hand passes "through" the fingers of your left hand and off the top of his penis, grasp his penis with your left hand and slide down its shaft. While your left hand is sliding down, move your right hand slightly away and back to the base of his penis. After your left hand slides down and away, repeat the upstroke with your right hand. While the upstroke is going on, your left hand returns to the head of his penis so its stroke can be repeated. Both hands move in oval-like shapes, and both move in either a clockwise or counter-clockwise direction. Of course, that direction can be reversed. Use a slow speed at first, then increase and/or vary the speed as appropriate.

Make A Tent

If you're looking for a simple but effective way to spice up masturbating him, simply drape the bed sheet over his penis while you stroke it. Just remember that you may need a clean sheet in the very near future. Satin sheets provide an extra-sensual variation.

Merry-Go-Round

Place your hands on either side of his cock as though you were about to Make a Snake (Trick 43). But instead of simply moving them back and forth, move them in circles, as though you were rolling a ball of clay. The circles go in the same direction (e.g., both clockwise), but one hand should be coming toward you as the other is moving away from you. (The up-and-down "horse" in the merry-go-round may be him.)

Climbing The Mountain

This masturbation game can drive a man absolutely nuts. (It was one of the most popular tricks from the original Tricks series). It's usually done with him lying on his back.

Sit or kneel comfortably either beside him or between his legs. Take his penis in one hand and gently, sensuously caress it for about ten seconds, then give it *one* quick up-and-down stroke. Repeat the sensuous caressing for about ten seconds – perhaps doing slow up-and-down strokes, perhaps doing other things that feel good to him – then give his penis *two* quick up-and-down strokes. Repeat the sensual caressing, then give *three* quick strokes. Then more caressing, followed by *four* quick strokes. Then more caressing, and *five* strokes. You get the idea. Continue to "climb the mountain" as long as you can.

One tip: the man may reach a point where his orgasm is becoming inevitable, and slow caressing might spoil it. He is therefore allowed to say (assuming he can still coherently speak) "keep going" *one time*, after which you give him only rapid strokes until he has an orgasm. He should climax within one minute. (If he doesn't, an appropriate pre-negotiated "penalty" should be administered.)

interlude: an adventure

lap dancing

Note from author: This essay was submitted by Trickster Andrew Conway. Although its length precluded including it as a regular trick, I liked it so much that I wanted to include it in the book somehow, so here it is:

In many strip clubs, dancers offer lap dances. The nude (or nearly nude) dancer squirms on the client's lap, allowing intimate sexual contact while stopping short of actual sex. The dancer tries to keep the client sexually aroused for as long as possible, close to orgasm but not actually coming, so he will keep paying for more dances.

There are strict rules about what is and is not allowed. The limits will vary with the local jurisdiction, the club and the dancer. In some clubs the client is not allowed to touch the dancer, in others he can grope all he likes so long as he does not stick his fingers in her pussy. Kissing and licking are generally forbidden. The lucky recipient should be fully clothed, and his cock should stay firmly zipped inside his pants. The dancer should wear high heeled shoes and sexy underwear (or perhaps nothing but the shoes). I would suggest that for home use the dancer decides in advance what the limits are to be, and makes these clear to the dancee. For instance, "You can touch me anywhere you like except my panties. No kissing, licking, or biting. Don't try and undress yourself or me. Now sit back and enjoy this."

Opinions may differ as to what makes a good lap dance, but let me tell you what I would like you to do if you were dancing on my lap.

Dim the lights. Put on some sexy music, fairly loud. Normally lap dancers time their dances by the song and will expect more money when each new song starts playing, but we can dispense with that at home. However, it would be a good idea if at the start of each song you ask me if I want more. It's all part of the tease.

First song:

I will be seated on a couch. (Some prefer the possibilities of a straight-backed chair, but I like the comfort of relaxing on a couch.) Spread my knees and stand between them, while you sway in time to the music. Caress your breasts and pussy through your underwear. Smile and pout. Take off your bra, and play with your bare breasts. Lean forward, and squeeze them together in front me. Let me bury my face in them for a couple of seconds, and then pull back. Let your hair drift across my face. Hold the back of the couch for balance while you rub your knee (gently!) on my crotch.

Second song:

Now turn around, and bend over. Gyrate your bottom in my face. I'd prefer you to be wearing a thong or G-string, but if you have bikini style panties on, pull them up into the crack of your ass for maximal buttock exposure. Spread your knees, and pull your panties to one side to give me a quick glimpse, then slide them back. Reach back between your legs and rub first your crotch and then mine. By now you should be able to feel a very hard cock through my pants.

Third song:

Push my legs together and straddle them with your legs. Now you finally get to sit on my lap, facing away from me. Support some of your weight on your hands, as you squirm your ass backwards and forwards. By now my hands will be on your body, caressing your thighs, your belly and your breasts. As I run my fingers over your nipples, lean back your head and growl in the back of your throat. If my hands stray to your panties, you can stop me breaking the limit by moving my hand away and saying, "No, not there," or even standing up and dancing away from me for a while if I persist. Remember to keep me wanting more.

Fourth song:

Kneel on the couch, facing towards me and straddling my legs. Grip the back of the couch for balance if you need to. Rub your crotch against mine. If you think I am getting too excited, kneel up a little and rub your breasts on my face. I'm going to be squeezing your ass and fondling your breasts. Respond to my pelvic thrusts by pulling away a little. Remember this is all about teasing.

Fifth song:

Remove your panties and repeat the fourth song. Whisper in my ear how hard my cock feels. By now, if you have been doing this properly, you should be covered in sweat. Tell me about that, too. Moan from time to time.

That's about as far as a dance will go even in the most liberal of strip clubs, but at home you may wish to start relaxing the limits at this point...

oral tricks

Whole books can be, and have been, written about the fine art of fellatio – a sexual exchange so commonplace today that it's hard to remember that it's been a matter of mere decades since it was illegal in most states, and considered perverse and immoral by many "God-fearing" Americans. Today, it holds an honored and well-deserved place on the menu of most sexually adventurous couples, both as an appetizer and as a main course. Here, you'll find some Tricksters' ideas for solving a few common problems, and some clever ways to make something as fabulous as fellatio even better (difficult though that may seem to imagine).

51 A Fistful of Fun

Grasp the penis just below its head in a firm but not tight fist. Take the head of his penis, above your fist, into your mouth. He can then thrust his penis through your fist into your mouth, creating the desired friction with his own motion.

Hookers' Trick #2

Many (if not most) men, while they're being fellated, like to come in their partner's mouth. Unfortunately, not everyone loves the taste of semen. My sources tell me that you won't taste it as much if you place your tongue over the head of his penis shortly before he comes, and I can tell you firsthand that it's difficult to detect any difference in sensation when this is done to you.

That Deep-Down Feeling

To control the depth to which he's going in your mouth, wrap one hand (or both, if needed) around his cock, as far back from the head as you want to let him in. That way his whole cock is being stimulated, and you only have to take in as much as you want. To give him that all-over wet feel, you can lick him all over first, or lube him with a flavored lube.

So Many Ways to Suck

A mistress of the art writes: "Fellatio done well includes a variety of sensations. The variations may be subtle, but there's at least two suction techniques you can use.

"Start off keeping your tongue firmly out of the way, in the bottom of your mouth. Don't use the tongue to create suction; let your cheeks and lips apply the pressure. Once you've got a good seal, begin to slide your mouth up and then down the shaft. Go slowly; the suction it takes to keep a mouth sealed can pull skin. Once you have that technique down, begin to use your tongue to create the suction. This frees the lips up quite a bit, making it easier to slide your mouth up and down the shaft while creating an entirely different suction pressure. When you reach the head, use your tongue to circle the coronal ridge without breaking suction. That may take some practice, but the results will be worth the effort.

"Experiment with alternating the types of suction, starting easy and working up. Gentle suction applied after firm suction carries far less impact."

Child's Play

Take just a small amount of his soft cock in your mouth and nurse on it, just like a baby would nurse on a bottle or a nipple.

That's Deep, Man

Want to take him deeper into your mouth? Try lying flat on your back on the bed, with your head over the edge so that it falls backward. Open your mouth and let him insert his penis into your mouth "upside-down." The stretch in your neck opens up your throat and may let you accept more of his penis than in more conventional positions.

Second Stage of the Booster Rocket

He may honestly feel that he's too tired that night to have sex, the poor dear. A few minutes of fellatio just may change his mind.

58
Peek-A-Boo

Men are notoriously visual creatures, and you can tease him with what you let him see – and what you don't let him see. If you have long hair, surround yourself with it during fellatio and only occasionally let him see his cock in your mouth, shimmering through a veil of hair.

59
Lick, Don't Swallow

Let's say that you are performing fellatio and your partner begins to ejaculate. You don't want to swallow his semen, and yet you also want to give him a very pleasurable orgasm. Try using the tip of your tongue to briskly lick along the underside of his penis, just at the junction of the shaft and the head. Continue doing this for nearly a minute.

He should have a very pleasant orgasm (trust me on this) and yet very little of his semen should get into your mouth. This technique can sometimes provide a very acceptable compromise between swallowing his semen and pulling your mouth away entirely.

60

Knock, Knock, Come In

Fellatio can often be enhanced by tapping the shaft of his penis with your fingers while your mouth works on its head. You can vary the tapping from light to firm, from occasional to regular, and in various rhythms.

61

A Palatable Suggestion

Many male Tricksters report that if they can feel the head of their cock on the roof of their partner's mouth, then it *really* feels like it's in their partner's mouth.

62

An Open-Faced Tongue Sandwich

Take his cock deep into your mouth. While holding it there, make your tongue flat and soft, then rub its flat surface in circles on the underside of his cock.

Blowing Hot and Cold

This Trick is deceptively simple, but nonetheless often highly effective. If you gently blow on something such as a penis or nipple from very close, your breath feels hot. If you back off about six to twelve inches and blow, your breath feels cold. Wetting the blown-upon object with your saliva increases both sensations. Hot and cold can be alternated to good effect. This can be combined well with masturbation and "regular" oral sex.

Ball And Socket

Take just the head of his penis in your mouth, then pivot your head in clockwise and counterclockwise circles (don't strain your neck).

65 Gag Gift

If you have a tendency to gag while performing fellatio, try breathing through your nose while his cock is in your mouth. You may find that doing so reduces the gagging considerably.

66 Channel Surfing

Just for an occasional treat, when he's channel surfing, let him keep on with that while you go down on him. It's interesting to see how long it will take for him to put down the remote.

Come Across The Ridge

When you are doing either manual or oral stimulation of your male partner and you want him to come to orgasm, make sure your strokes of his penis go all the way up the shaft and slip over the ridge of the penis. The area on the lower edge of this ridge (it's called the corona) is where the nerve endings live that when stimulated result most easily in orgasm. In many men, you have to stimulate this particular area to produce an orgasm – or *avoid* stimulating this area to not produce one.

Don't Choke In The Clutch

If you're having trouble suppressing your gag reflex during fellatio, try using some sore-throat spray a few minutes beforehand – perhaps even gargling with it a bit. The cool, numbing sensation that results should help you cope a bit better. Of course, if you insert his penis very soon after you spray your throat, he'll receive some of the same "benefits."

Depth Charge

During fellatio, relax your tongue, even move it a bit forward, and you may be able to take him deeper into your mouth.

Making Friends

Hold the penis in your mouth for a long time, just to show that you like this part of his body.

Hooker's Trick #3

Many men like to watch. Therefore, when asked to perform fellatio, many hookers position themselves so their customer can see his cock entering their mouth.

Footnote: If you feel like teasing him, position yourself so that he *can't* see his cock entering your mouth.

72

Here He Comes, And I'm Glad

Many men love the idea of coming in a woman's mouth, but are uncertain about how they'll be received. Saying (as best you can) "uh huh, uh huh" as he's reaching his orgasm lets him know you're happy that he's about to come in your mouth.

73

Cold Tongue

Take a medium-sized bite of crushed ice, then give him a blow job. He'll shiver… in ecstasy.

74

A Bit of The Bubbly

When performing fellatio, stopping occasionally to place a sip of champagne in your mouth and then reinserting his penis can liven things up wonderfully. (A soft drink can provide a nice, non-alcoholic alternative.)

Huff-N-Puff

Give him a literal blow job. Take his cock in your mouth and blow, either with or without a seal created by your lips.

Hum Job

Humming while using your mouth on various parts of your lover's body can add a light, silly, and often erotic tone. Depending on the situation, humming certain songs can be fun. "Happy Birthday" has a cult following.

Terra Incognita

The perineum – the space behind his scrotum but in front of his anus – is rich with nerves and often very sensitive to touch. Try running your tongue lengthwise or back and forth along the little ridge of flesh there and you may be surprised at his dramatic reaction. (If you're apprehensive about playing in this area, try it when he's fresh out of the shower or tub.)

78 Tea for Two

Temperature play is a favorite oral sex trick. One of the simplest yet most effective variants is to simply keep a cup of hot liquid by the bed: coffee, tea, or plain hot water. One of my most informed sources of information regarding fellatio said that, of all her methods, this was the simplest, easiest to control, and evoked the most response.

79 The Crown of Thorns

This trick can be extremely intense, perhaps too intense for some men, but it can really work for others. As always, feedback is essential. Take his cock into your mouth and, just behind its head, gently bite down on it. Now use your teeth to stimulate his cock. Bite down "just a little" and then rock your head from side to side, nod your head up and down, swivel your head in circles, and so forth. To add extra spice, you can also from time to time flick the head of his penis with your tongue.

Hooker's Trick #4

Note to my readers: This is almost certainly the trick that received the most attention out of the entire original Tricks series. Enjoy!

A time-honored cat house specialty is the Crème de Menthe blow job. Its unusual color, minty odor, and hot/cool sensation (along with its regular benefits) have helped prostitutes pay the rent for many years.

You put a teaspoon of the green variety in your mouth and then touch his penis to your lips. Open your mouth very slightly and let the liquor out. Make sure he can see the green spread. Once the green has spread over his cock, open your mouth until it's open slightly wider than his cock – a bit farther than you usually would. Lower your mouth way down over his penis, with your lips close to but not touching it, and blow out. After that, with your lips still not quite touching, suck in air (rather forcefully) as you raise your head up the shaft of his penis. This creates an exquisite, cool sensation. Repeat as desired.

Footnote #1: The liquor also feels good on his testicles. Footnote #2: You can also fan his liquor-coated cock with a pretty, feathered fan to good effect.

Warning: My source for this Trick cautioned me that the alcohol is likely to burn too much for it to work well during cunnilingus.

68 tricks

interlude 2:
another adventure

hot sex

Menthol is a chemical substance found in a lot of over-the-counter pharmaceuticals such as toothpaste, mouthwash, sports rubs, chest rubs and so on. Lovers who like to add a little intensity to their lovemaking sometimes include it in their play for its ability to create intense sensations when applied to the skin, sensations which are usually felt either as heat or as "chilled heat." A similar substance, capsicum, is found in foodstuffs such as hot sauce and in a few sports rubs, and is felt purely as heat; it is generally considered more intense but is sometimes also used in play. A few people also enjoy experimenting with cinnamon oil, wasabi and other "hot" foods. All these kinds of products can be used to spice up fellatio or cunnilingus, or as a masturbation lubricant, either solo or in addition to your regular lube of choice. Their labels will tell you whether or not they contain menthol and/or capsicum.

Most of these products are not designed, intended, or recommended for internal use (except for the foods, which are intended for use in the mouth only). Using them inside the genitals or anus is not recommended. I have heard of some lunatics attempting to use them for penetration, but in most cases such usage was more painful than they could stand. These substances can also upset the natural biological balance of such areas.

A very small amount of "hot sex" can, in some cases, be applied to the clitoris to make female masturbation more intense, but please be careful. Remember, these substances are not intended for internal use, and it feels much "hotter" on mucous membranes. Ladies, I suggest you try this on your own before involving another person. Menthol-containing cough drops might be used during cunnilingus, but please note the above warnings carefully. These substances must be used cautiously. Whereas other tricks are spices, "hot sex" qualifies as, well, red-hot pepper. Using a *very* small amount may spice things up nicely. Using too much can cause genuine agony.

Start slowly and with small amounts when using a "hot sex" cream. It's often wise to dilute it with another lubricant, at least at first. Never use the extra-strength brand of anything until you've used the regular strength brand successfully several times. Understand that gels can be *much* hotter than creams.

"Hot sex" substances may take up to five minutes for the effects of a given "dose" to be fully felt, so take your time about adding more. One dose is usually felt for about twenty minutes, but this can vary considerably from person to person and from product to product. Such substances applied to the scrotum are usually felt sooner and feel hotter than the same substance applied to the penis.

A Few Cautions

There is a very slight possibility of your choking if you perform fellatio while holding a foreign object, such as an ice cube, peppermint candy, or cough drop, in your mouth. Therefore, never attempt such a trick while even slightly intoxicated, and make sure you know how to do the Heimlich maneuver on yourself. (Using the back of a chair helps a lot.)

Many of these substances are oil-based, and thus should be avoided in situations that require condoms and other latex barriers.

If you use these substances to masturbate a man, a considerable amount will get on your hand as well as his cock. Because the skin of your hand is much thicker than the skin of his penis, it may take time for you to feel this.

"Burning Hands Syndrome" can develop an hour or more after the session. You might therefore wear latex or vinyl gloves when playing with "hot sex," especially capsicum.

Be careful about combining these substances with abrasion. Skin that has been scraped, such as by fingernails, will be considerably less able to tolerate such play.

Menthol in particular leaves a distinct smell in the air. It's a good idea to use it only in well-ventilated areas if the lingering smell might be a problem.

"Overdoses"

It's easy to add more of whatever substance you're using, but it's very difficult to remove what you've already applied. If you do have a "hot sex overdose," you can usually wash it off by using cold running water and lots of soap. Applying large amounts of shampoo and then washing it off works especially well. Very liberal amounts of the astringent called witch hazel also wash it off. (Your drugstore carries it.) You can also "cool things down" by rubbing on generous amounts of petroleum jelly or an oil-based cream. (Be sure you don't use a chest rub!) I haven't personally tested it, but I'm told that cold cream works well. Physically cooling the area seems to help.

You might consider deliberately creating an overdose in order to test these various cool-down methods. That way, in an actual "emergency," you'll have a clearer idea of what works (and what doesn't). Understand that different people may respond better to different cooling methods.

Don't combine "hot sex" play with bondage until you, your partner, and the substance in question are well acquainted. An overdose is especially likely to occur during the first one or two times you use a given substance with a new partner. If they get overdosed and need to run to the shower, they'll need to be able to run there *now*.

I don't recommend using this kind of play with a new partner unless they (and you) are already highly experienced in its use. It's too easy for things to go wrong and perhaps harm your budding relationship. Use this only for self-play or with someone you already know well. It would be a good idea to use a particular lubricant on yourself several times before you ask a partner to use it on you.

Because most of these substances "burn" for about twenty minutes after being applied (some brands burn longer), and because this feeling may be seriously unpleasant if no longer accompanied by sexual arousal, it's both wise and compassionate to wait for its sensations to fade to a very low level before bringing your partner to orgasm.

As you can see, "hot sex" is one of the more serious tricks, with a steeper learning curve than most. Use it properly, though, and you can add an enormous amount of intensity and pleasure to your lovemaking.

74 interlude

enhanced tricks

These days, while the bodies of the lovers are a good place to start for great sex, sometimes more is needed (or wanted). Of course, safer sex – unless you're in a completely monogamous relationship, or one in which you and your lover have agreed to use barrier protection with everybody except one another – mandates the use of condoms and other barriers, so a certain amount of "equipment" is required right there. Add to that the use of vibrators and other sex toys – and more and more men are discovering that these can add a whole new dimension to their sex lives as well as those of their women friends – and the nightstand drawer has gotten deeper. And finally, there's the whole category of "wild stuff": while this book isn't specifically kink-oriented, even couples whose sex lives are relatively "vanilla" sometimes like to experiment with a bit of bondage, role-play or more intense sensation.

So this section is all about "enhanced tricks": ways to make your safer sex more fun… new and different ways to use your sex toys… ways to bring just a little bit of fudge ripple or pecan pistachio into your vanilla sex life. They're generally arranged from tame to wild. Have fun!

81 A Little Dab'll'Do Ya

One of the single simplest things you can do to improve the sensation of condom use is to add a single drop of water-based lubricant to the inside of the tip of the condom before you roll it on. The lubricant enables the condom to move more freely over the skin of your penis, as well as improving the way heat is conducted through the material of the condom, so you can feel your partner's body heat more naturally. Only one drop, though – use too much lube and it might get down the shaft of the condom and make it too slippery to stay put on your cock.

82 The Fashionably Baggy Fit

One particular style of condom comes with a "pouch" around the head of the penis, which is the most sensitive part on many men. Some men prefer this style of condom for intercourse, finding that it greatly enhances their sensation by creating the greatest possible movement against this nerve-rich area.

Search And Rescue

Pubic hair, as well as hair from other areas, occasionally ends up in your mouth, and this can be a major irritation and distraction. I've had excellent results in removing such hair by using an ordinary toothbrush.

Watering Can

Water-based lubes are seeing much wider use than they previously did. (They're compatible with condom usage, whereas oil-based lubricants can dissolve a condom.) Unfortunately, water-based lubricants can "dry out" more quickly than do oil-based lubes. Tricksters thus often keep a small, fliptop bottle of water close to their small, fliptop bottle of lube. One useful way to accomplish this is to tape or glue the two bottles together. This is an almost optimally handy arrangement.

The Magical Vibrating Weenie

Grab that vibe, guy, and hold it against the base of your cock while she performs fellatio on you. Why should she be the only one to have vibrator fun?

Fashion Statement

An undershirt, preferably an old, very soft one, can make an excellent cloth for wiping yourself or your partner off during and after sex. Placing any long, cylindrical parts inside the neck, sleeves, or bottom of the shirt works particularly well.

Alternative Approaches

It's possible that he doesn't want to use a condom for intercourse because he has greater difficulty reaching orgasm while he's wearing one. An alternative approach is to have intercourse for a while with him wearing one, then remove the condom and bring him to orgasm with your hands and/or mouth.

Note: Fellatio without a barrier is certainly safer than intercourse without a barrier as regards AIDS and some other sexually transmitted diseases, but is risky as regards herpes and several others. You and your partner must discuss these risks and make your own decisions about whether barrier-free fellatio is OK for you. If unwanted pregnancy is your main concern, however, fellatio can be a great solution.

A Vibrator Built For Two

Several Tricksters mentioned that if the woman uses a strong vibrator on the front of her vulva, below her pubic bone – sometimes called the external g-spot – during doggy style intercourse, he can feel the vibrations, too. One lady mentioned, "This is a great, non-threatening way to get him used to including the vibrator in mutual play because there's also something in it for him."

Cape of Good Hope

One of the many excellent tricks contributed by "The Retired Courtesan" is as follows: "I have more than once arrived at a man's house dressed in a big, ankle-length cape. Then I invite him to open (or unzip) the cape and underneath I am either naked or wearing something very seductive."

Cheek To Cheek

Take his penis into your mouth, then apply a vibrator to your cheek. Move the vibrator sensuously from one cheek to the other. Touch it to your lips. Apply it to the point of your chin. Turn your head so that the head of his penis makes a bulge in one of your cheeks and apply the vibrator to that bulge.

Donna Reed Lives!

A very experienced lady Trickster writes, "I love old-fashioned housewife's aprons. Sometimes it's fun to announce it's time to clean house and take everything off *but* the apron. Feather dusters can be fun in this game, too. My partner has had his nose and toes, and other parts, dusted quite a few times in the course of house cleaning. Usually stops the clean-up though. Probably explains the condition of our house."

Hair Heaven

If you have long hair, you can use it to whip your lover. Your hair can feel wonderfully sensuous on his chest, back, and other body areas. One caution: Keep clear of his face. A lock of your hair swiped across his bare eyeballs can, to say the least, spoil the mood. Swing your hair back and forth, sideways, and in other directions. (Don't hurt your neck.) If it's long enough, hold it in your hand and use it. Women who have very long hair can often combine this trick with her-on-top intercourse.

An alternative: One lady Trickster who wears her hair Marine-buzz short tells me she enjoys using its plushy texture as a sex toy, brushing her soft head over her lover's tender bits.

Nature is a Mother

Here's *the* big trick for sex on the beach, in the woods, and so forth. Bring a blanket! Various bits of "Mother Nature" have a way of getting in the most intimate places, at the most awkward times, unless you bring something, preferably something *wide*, to lie on.

94 Imaginary Bondage

One Trickster writes: "Take your partner's hands and feet and put them where you want them, and tell him he is now tied in that position. My boyfriend and I do this and he gets so into it he won't move until I tell him he can, even after we're done!"

By the way, this is a great, non-threatening way to begin experimenting with bondage games should you and your partner feel so inclined.

95 Sock It To Me

Many men like to slip a sock over their penis while they masturbate (or when they're being masturbated by a partner). It does a wonderful job of catching the semen in a non-messy way. Different textures have their fans, as do different colors!

96 Vibes for Guys

Vibrators aren't just "girl stuff," fellas. Try using a vibrator on various parts of your genitals – many male Tricksters enjoy the vibration on their penis (particularly on the underside just below the head), their perineum, and their anus. If it's her vibrator you're using, or if you want to use it on someone else later, cover it carefully with a condom, rubber glove, or plastic wrap, or put plastic wrap over the part of you that you're stimulating.

97 Ooooh, Baby, Baby

A mischievous lady Trickster suggests taking a baby's teething ring — "a nice big round one" — and slipping it behind both the penis and testicles to form a cock ring. To spice this one up a bit, you can either warm it up or cool it down before slipping it on.

Thuck Me, Baby!

Touch a small, battery operated vibrator to the underside of your tongue during oral sex, thus turning your tongue into a vibrating sex toy.

Men Often Make Passes…

While sex is usually about increasing intimacy, one way to add a bit of spice is to sometimes make it a bit more impersonal. A highly experienced lady Trickster achieves this by wearing mirrored sunglasses. She particularly likes wearing these when playing domination/submission games with her lover, but they can work well during more conventional lovemaking too.

Frothing at the Mouth

Take a sip of champagne or a soft drink, hold it in your mouth, and insert his penis. (This trick itself can be very intense.) Now touch a vibrator to your cheek and notice his reaction.

101

Cubes and Balls

Put an ice cube (one with no sharp edges or corners) in your hand, and apply your hand to his well-lubricated penis. Now touch a vibrator to the base of his penis while you masturbate its head. (If you're using a plug-in vibrator, be very careful that no part of the vibrator gets wet except for its head.)

102

Three's Company

If she enjoys the sensation of wearing a butt plug, he may find that having it in her during intercourse makes her vagina feel tighter and more interesting.

103   Dental Hygiene

You can definitely make fellatio more interesting for him (as if it weren't already interesting enough!) by placing some toothpaste in your mouth before going down on him. Pepsodent™ has something of a cult following, as does Close-up™.

104   Chocolate Kiss

Fellatio can be made more interesting and pleasurable for the giver if she places a small piece of chocolate in her mouth while she's doing it. Of course, she may need more than one piece.

105   Two Can Play At This Game

During woman-on-top intercourse, if she uses a strong vibrator to stimulate her anal area, she can simultaneously use it to vibrate his balls. This game can be intensified by adding a butt plug for her and/or a cock ring for him.

106

Just A Pinch For Seasoning

Many a man's orgasm can be enhanced by pinching his scrotum (not his actual testicles) as he has an orgasm. The welcome degree of pressure can range from very light to distinctly strong.

107

Lana's Point

A friend of mine, a sexually dominant woman, delights in delaying her partner's orgasm by requiring that he keep his toes pointed up, not curled under, while she provides whatever kind of sexual stimulation she's in the mood to offer. As most men instinctively curl their toes when they're approaching orgasm, the distraction is a mischievous and intense way of prolonging the inevitable.

108 Outlook Hot and Wet

Apply some "warming" lotion (the kind supplied by vendors of adult products) to his penis – the type that feels warmer when you blow on it. (Not Ben Gay™ or something similar.) Now put one or two ice cubes, or some crushed ice, in your mouth and fellate him.

109 The Painless Whipping

Perhaps the idea of one of you whipping the other on their back or butt has come up, but you're not too sure of how to go about it, plus you're not really sure that either you or your partner wants to receive a lot of pain. In such a situation, try using an ordinary pillowcase as an exploratory toy. Such a pillowcase can be used either by simply holding it in the hand by one end or by first rolling it up.

The Bald and the Beautiful

With his prior permission for all of the following, first tie him down securely, then clip his pubic hair closely and carefully with a small sharp pair of scissors. Slowly and sensually shave his pubic area (using warm suds and water, a towel, several disposable razors, and occasional touches of tongue), then caress him with warm sweet oil. The sensation on skin that's never been bare before can drive him wild. Important note: he will be very itchy for several days afterward. Regular scrubbing with a loofah or Buf-Puf™ will help reduce ingrown hairs, antihistamine cream will help reduce itching, and boxers rather than briefs will reduce irritation, but some of it he'll just have to live with. I suspect he'll agree that it will have been worth it.

111 Juggling Balls

Encircle the top of his scrotum with your thumb and forefinger. Squeeze this ring together until it's snug and his testicles are "trapped" below it, then slowly pull down until the skin of his scrotum is pulled tight over his testicles. (See Trick 35.) Now apply your vibrator to the tight-skinned sack. (Note: pulling down too quickly, too long, or too hard could cause damage; be sure to get feedback from him.)

112 Getting Spicy

It's reliably reported to me that fellatio can be enhanced by using cinnamon oil as a penis lubricant. (Be sure you read "Interlude 2" before attempting this trick.) Many men find straight cinnamon oil too intense. You can dilute the oil with something tamer like plain vegetable oil, or try cinnamon leaf oil, a milder version. The woman who told me about this trick remarked, "There are so many different ways to give head that it just blows me away!"

interlude 3:
yet another adventure

the five "shuns" of anal play

The anal region has a good supply of nerve endings. Skillful anal play can be very rewarding, both physically and psychologically. Reports of orgasm from anal play alone are not rare. Still, this activity should not be done hurriedly or carelessly. The anus and rectum are not built to accommodate insertion. While fingers, butt plugs, dildoes, vibrators, anal beads, and other items have all been inserted successfully, this area of erotic play requires a high level of awareness.

Successful anal play can be looked at in terms of the five "tions" (shuns). They are, in the approximate order you'll need them: information, protection, lubrication, relaxation, and communication.

Information

The receptive person should tell their partner about their past experiences (or lack thereof) regarding anal sex, particularly any problems that have occurred. They should also mention any anal or rectal problems they have, such as hemorrhoids, fissures, an enlarged prostate, or more serious medical conditions. People with heart disease should know that heavy bearing down, during anal play or during a bowel movement, can slow the rate and force of their heartbeat, occasionally to zero. Use appropriate caution and seek medical consultation as necessary.

Protection

Disease can be transmitted in both directions during anal play. For this reason, barrier usage is very strongly recommended. Dildoes, plugs, vibrators and penises should be covered with condoms. Hands and fingers should be covered with gloves. Toys and hands should be cleaned afterwards.

Lubrication

The vagina and the mouth supply their own lubrication; the rectum does not. While the vagina sometimes needs extra lubrication, the rectum essentially always does. In general, heavier, more gel-like lubricants tend to work better than lighter, more liquid ones. Nowadays, water-soluble lubricants are preferred over oil-soluble lubricants, particularly if latex condoms and/or gloves are being used. Colored or scented lubricants should probably be avoided. Remember: "Lube early, lube often."

Relaxation

While erotic fiction contains many depictions of a person hating yet loving having something shoved suddenly and deeply into their rectum by an uncaring, dominant partner, the reality is far different. They'll probably just hate it, and it may cause them serious injury.

The anus has two rings of sphincter muscle: the external and the internal. The internal takes longer to relax. Start very gently and ease in only one finger. (Placing a cotton ball in the fingertip of your glove can help eliminate any "sharp" feeling, particularly if you have long fingernails.) Use lots of lube, don't move the finger around too much, and pay close attention. You may actually feel the sphincter relax. When you can move one finger in and out easily, add more lube and try slowly inserting a second finger. I recommend you not insert a vibrator or dildo until you can easily move two fingers all the way in and out. Having this done to you will teach you a great deal about how to do it to someone else.

Communication

Successful anal penetration requires feedback. Even a small variation in pressure, location, depth, or angle can make a major difference in how well the play goes. The receiving partner must communicate these matters clearly and promptly to the inserting person so necessary adjustments can be made. Above all, the receiving partner shouldn't "tough it out" in silence in order to please their lover. If something feels wrong, it almost undoubtedly is wrong and needs prompt correction. Anal play is *not* the time for the receptive partner to take a "stoic heroic" approach. Ongoing communication and adjustment are essential.

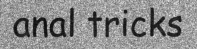

Many heterosexual men are intrigued by the idea of anal play, but have been given a lot of erroneous ideas that anal play is somehow the exclusive province of gay men. Nothing could be further from the truth. Every man has a prostate gland, and many men, straight and gay alike, find stimulation of the prostate to be sexually arousing – nothing about anal play is inherently "gay" (unless, of course, you're doing it with another man). If you've been avoiding this nerve-rich and exciting part of your body because of something someone told you years ago, you have a treat in store: read on!

113

Easy In

The initial entry of anal insertion is often the most uncomfortable part for the receptive partner. This discomfort can often be minimized by holding the plug or dildo stationary and letting him "back" onto it at his own pace. Entry can also be made easier if he bears down (as he does when having a bowel movement) while the object is being inserted. Tricksters who enjoy using butt plugs on themselves often set the plug down, business end up, on a chair or toilet seat cover and gradually lower themselves onto it.

No Oww Is Good Oww

If he's new to the sensations of anal sex, it can be difficult to tell which sensations are "right," and which ones mean something's wrong. In general, mild sensations of stretching, *mild* pain and burning, and feelings of having to defecate are all normal, especially at first. Any sharp pain, intense burning, or pain that lasts beyond the first couple of minutes is a sign that something isn't right. Most people have an instinctive sense of the difference between "good pain" and "bad pain" – if he's feeling the second one, stop, back off, try a smaller insertable or more lubrication or more relaxation, or simply move on to another activity and try again another day. Getting all goal-oriented isn't a good idea during any kind of sex, but most especially during anal sex.

Fore and Aft

During fellatio, try a little anal stimulation on him. One sex worker I interviewed noted, "Some guys don't like this at all, but most guys I know do (and as a pro, I talk to a *lot* of guys)." Try anything from light stroking of the anus to actual insertion of a finger. (Don't forget lube!)

Feverish Lust

If your partner is willing to experiment with anal play but is feeling extremely nervous about the whole idea, a wise Trickster recommends starting with an ordinary rectal thermometer. It's just about the least invasive item you can use. Of course, you should be gentle, use lube, and don't put it in too far (be sure you can keep a firm grip on the body of the thermometer with at least two fingers and your thumb).

Burn, Baby, Burn

Much as you and your honey might enjoy anal play, it can sometimes leave unpleasant smells in the bedroom. Burning a pretty candle on a nearby nightstand, scented or not as you prefer, can greatly reduce this problem.

Self-Help Manual

This is a very simple trick, but it can be of great importance. Many Tricksters find that they can explore anal insertion play much more easily and productively if they insert the object themselves rather than having someone else manipulate it.

It's All In The Timing

Many Tricksters enjoy anal play, but are grossed out by small amounts of fecal matter on (animate or inanimate) toys. Right after a bowel movement may be a good time to do anal penetration play. If that timing isn't convenient, you may want to try a ready-made drugstore enema about half an hour to an hour before you play.

120 Slow In, Slow Out

Once again, this is a very simple trick, but it can be of great importance. Be sure to remove your anal toy slowly and carefully. Yanking it out feels unpleasant and could cause injury.

121 Fingers First

While many men like to be anally penetrated by a woman wearing a strap-on dildo, it may not be smart to rush directly into this activity. A wise woman who has played this game with many different partners advises first inserting some gloved fingers. Feel for any unusual bumps, roughness, or swelling, and watch for any blood.

If the recipient can take two fingers, then try using a small hand-held dildo on him. If that goes well, *then* you can try moving on to the strap-on type – probably in another session. More than any other kind of play, anal play rewards patient players.

The Most Intimate Touch

"Rimming" – tonguing, licking or kissing the anal area – is a form of sex play that invokes many taboos, and does involve some health risks. Yet many couples find it intriguing and, with proper care and preparation, highly enjoyable.

If you'd like to add this special trick to your repertoire, it's best to do so with a steady monogamous partner, or to use a barrier of latex (a dental dam works well, or you can unroll an unlubricated condom and cut down one side to make a flat piece of latex) or a piece of household plastic wrap between the giver's tongue and the recipient's anus. Many couples also like to shower, bathe or hot-tub together beforehand. The use of a flavored lubricant, or a good-tasting oil (see Trick 46), might be enjoyable as well.

Then – explore. Lick, stroke, probe, flutter. See what feels good, better, best. How often do you have a whole, brand-new area of the body to explore like this?

That Deep-Down Slippery Feeling

It can sometimes be difficult to get lube *inside* the rectum, where you need it for activities that involve in-and-out thrusting – the sphincter muscles scrape it off on its way in. A clever Trickster suggests using the type of plungers sold with vaginal spermicidal jelly.

Push out the jelly using the plunger mechanism and wash the empty syringe. Then "reload" the syringe with your lube of choice – many folks prefer thicker lube for anal play – insert it into the rectum, press the plunger, and you're ready to go. If he starts to feel a burning or raw sensation later in your play, simply repeat.

Kneesy Easy

He may have an easier time accepting anal insertion if he's on his back with his legs and knees in the air. (He can hold them up with his hands, or prop them on your shoulders.)

125 Come Hither

Once you get your finger into his rectum, stroke his prostate. Turn the palm of your hand towards the front of his body, then hook your finger down in a "come here" gesture to see if he will "go there."

And the Most Important Trick of All...

Have fun. Sex is – or should be – about pleasure, intimacy, connection, and warmth. If you're so hung up on technique that you're not enjoying yourself, you're missing the point. Relax, touch, open yourself up to giving and receiving pleasure, and you'll be back on track in no time.

Enjoy yourselves!

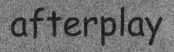

on sex, risk, probability, and decision-making

Having sex has always been dangerous. Vaginal intercourse has almost always involved at least a minimal risk of unwanted pregnancy. Most kinds of sex have always carried the possibility of acquiring an incurable, fatal disease. The big specter used to be syphilis – but about 20 years ago, AIDS emerged, and having sex suddenly became a lot more dangerous than it had been for quite some time. The reemergence of a fatal, incurable, sexually transmitted disease has once again changed the very fabric of how we live and will continue to change it for decades.

Moreover, we now know a lot more about sexually transmitted diseases that can have short-term and long-term effects on health and relationships: herpes, chlamydia, genital warts, and dozens more. AIDS is at the top of many sexually active people's worry lists, but it's far from being their only concern.

People want to know how they can have sex and yet protect themselves. Various authorities respond with this or that regimen. Some regimens are excellent; some are half-baked, or so demanding that many people, daunted by unrealistic advice, throw up their hands and abandon the whole idea of safer sex.

What I don't think is made clear enough to those seeking information is that essentially all of this is a matter of probabilities. No complication occurs 100% of the time, and no protective measure is

100% effective. It's all a case of shifting the odds. Granted, in many cases the odds can and should be shifted, but we need to make it clearer to people than we do that it's still a matter of probability. We see some signs of this shift in the emergence of the term "safer sex" to replace the somewhat misleading term "safe sex."

Early in the AIDS crisis, when the modes of disease transmission were less well understood than they are today, various authorities advocated nothing less than "total body fluid isolation" rules. Bedrooms all over America began to resemble hospital "protective isolation" wards.

Today, certain practices – particularly fellatio without ejaculation and cunnilingus – are believed to be somewhat less risky than previously thought. (Unprotected anal sex is considerably *more* risky than previously thought.) Unfortunately, no authority can recommend less than total body fluid isolation without becoming vulnerable to accusations of reckless irresponsibility by their more conservative peers. They therefore keep silent even though they might like to speak up.

And, to be fair, these more conservative peers have some merit in what they say. While the odds seem sharply against it, you most definitely can become infected with the virus that causes AIDS by performing only a single act of sex with an HIV-positive person.

Add into this mess the fact that the usual medical experiments to study infectious disease cannot, for ethical reasons, be conducted, plus the new strains of virus that are emerging, and you have a genuinely murky situation. As a finishing touch, add in the numerous personal, economic, social, political, and religious influences. The situation's clarity now drops to near zero.

So what do you do? Stop and think. Ask various authorities for information. Ask them (and yourself) how reliable and complete is the information on which they're basing their decisions and recommendations. Be sure to consider any possible hidden agendas, particularly any political or religious agendas, this authority may have.

Have you had an AIDS antibody test? This is one of the most responsible steps you can take. If you've had any unsafe contacts, have you had a test since then? Do you really understand what information such a test does and does not provide? Has the person you're considering having sex with had such a test? How reliable is their answer likely to be? Many, many people will lie right to your face if doing so will get you to have sex with them, particularly if their chance seems close.

As it stands now, masturbating your partner seems very safe, and a skillfully administered hand job can be one of the most intense sexual experiences possible. Make sure your hands have no open sores or hangnails, keep them away from your eyes and mucous membranes, and you're almost as safe as you can get. I personally have never heard of anyone getting infected or becoming pregnant from masturbating or being masturbated by their partner.

Unprotected oral sex seems relatively safe. Pregnancy is almost unheard of, and it's been reliably documented that saliva helps neutralize the AIDS virus. Still, some risk is involved. Please understand clearly that gonorrhea, syphilis, herpes, and other diseases can be transmitted this way (in both directions). Furthermore, the risk of getting AIDS, while small, does exist, and grows larger if the man ejaculates in his partner's mouth.

Unprotected vaginal sex is, of course, definitely risky. The risk of unplanned pregnancy and sexually transmitted disease is almost always present. Please be very, very careful about how and with whom you have vaginal intercourse.

Unprotected receptive anal sex seems to be, in terms of getting AIDS, the riskiest form of sex you can have these days. (The active role is not risk-free either.) A physician told me that the odds of getting infected by having a single act of unprotected, receptive anal sex with an HIV+ partner are a staggering one chance in three.

It should also be mentioned here that several STDs, notably herpes and genital warts, cannot be reliably prevented simply by using condoms. Contagious lesions sometimes form on parts of the genitals not protected by condoms, such as the pubic mound, scrotum and perineum. And "asymptomatic shedding" of the virus can also transmit disease even when no lesions are present.

Choosing which acts you'll participate in definitely helps shift the odds in your favor. A condom, provided it's used properly, adds considerable protection. Dental dams and latex or nitrile gloves play crucial roles.

There is no such thing as risk-free sex. Still, as with driving a car, flying a plane, or swimming, you can reduce the odds to a level where most people would consider the risk acceptable. You, of course, must decide where that level is for you. (Whatever you do, don't let another person make this decision for you.) Remember, nothing is 100%

dangerous and nothing is 100% safe. Also remember that STD clinics, pregnancy crisis centers, and AIDS wards are filled with people who insisted on blinding themselves to the full extent of the risks they took.

We live in an age where 60 seconds of clear thinking about what is proper sexual behavior for you can add 60 years to your life.

oops! - or, accidents happen

Before I start talking about strategies to employ when things go wrong, something to think about is where you'd go if this happened to you. Such incidents may not be something you want on your regular, permanent medical record. A visit to a local free clinic, women's clinic, or other resource may be more appropriate. Your local erotic boutique or SM-oriented leather store may be able to give you the name of a discreet, sex-positive physician. If you have a sex-positive, discreet friend who is a physician, nurse, paramedic, chiropractor, or other type of medical person, you may be able to get advice and/or a referral from them. Also, a sympathetic physician may be found by contacting local sexuality-related organizations such as clubs for gay men, lesbians, bisexuals, transgendered people, or SM folks. You may not have to give your real name, but please be open regarding medical information and pay your bill if at all possible. It is very wise to have your "Plan B" doctor lined up ahead of time. Trying to find such a person while under the stress of an urgent situation can be very difficult.

Sexuality author and educator Race Bannon maintains a list of physicians, chiropractors, therapists and other professionals who offer sexually nonjudgmental services; check it out at *www.bannon.com/kap*. Also, Dr. Charles Moser has written an excellent book, called "Health Care Without Shame: A Handbook for the Sexually Diverse and Their Caregivers," that will help you organize your thoughts around this issue.

What to Do When a Trick Bombs

Each person has their own unique physical and emotional pattern of erotic responsiveness. Among other things, that means every now and then a Trick that has always worked well on partners before may utterly turn off a new partner. The key phrase for handling this situation is "show compassion for everyone involved, including yourself."

If what you did *really* turned your partner off, try not to take it personally. (You wouldn't be human if you didn't take it somewhat personally, but try not to buy into that too deeply.) Remember, each person has their own pattern, and you can never completely know what that pattern looks like. Give them a brief apology, if that seems appropriate, then do what you can to move on to something else. There is probably little to be gained by stopping to argue or debate the point in depth, particularly right then. Save discussions for later.

On the other hand, if your partner starts to do something that really doesn't work for you, please diplomatically let them know that as soon as you can. Being "polite" in this situation may only allow your displeasure to build to uncontrollable levels. Speak up (courteously, please) as soon as possible. Remember, this is almost undoubtedly not willful misconduct on their part. They are probably doing it in an attempt, however misguided, to arouse you.

Speak up, but give them the benefit of the doubt, especially if this partner is relatively new.

What to Do When a Toy Gets "Lost"

Occasionally, a toy, condom or other item will drift up out of reach inside the vagina or the anus. This is rarely a medical emergency, but it's usually uncomfortable and can be dangerous if the toy stays in there long enough to block normal functioning or to build up a bacterial overload.

Toys lost in the vagina are less of an emergency. The vagina is a closed system (except during childbirth); the toy has no place to go. The rectum, on the other hand, is not a closed system and objects without a wide flange at their base can sometimes go in so far that they cannot be grasped with fingers.

If this does happen, keep in mind that the item will almost undoubtedly pass back out naturally and on its own before long. The natural peristaltic action of the bowel will prevent the item from working its way farther up. There's no need to mount a dramatic rescue operation. Above all, don't do anything that hurts. The item should appear no later than the next bowel movement. Assuming a squatting position, as opposed to the usual sitting position, may help pass the object.

(Caution: mild to moderate bearing down is probably OK. Hard straining could damage the rectal passage and, particularly if the individual has a heart condition, could possibly slow the heartbeat or even precipitate a cardiac arrest.)

You might be able to reach the item with a fingertip. If so, you may be able to ease it down until you can grasp it and (gently, slowly) extract it. One major caution: be careful not to push the item farther in. Sitting or standing in a upright position, or walking around for a while, may help the item work its way back down to where you can reach it.

Inserting an ounce or two of additional lubricant into the rectum may also help. At this point, a more liquid lubricant (such as mineral oil) is probably better. Careful use of an enema bulb or turkey baster can help ensure that the lubricant goes into the rectum. (See Trick 123 for another alternative.) He should lie on his left side as the lubricant is inserted and for several minutes thereafter, then sit, stand, or walk. A few don'ts:

- No enemas, please. Large volumes of water are not what the intestine needs just now. Among other things, the water may push the object further in, where it can really get stuck.

- No stimulant or irritant-type laxatives such as senna, bisacodyl, or castor oil.

A few possible options:

- Simply waiting is often a very rational strategy. There is a good chance that the item will pass out naturally. (If it isn't passed with the next bowel movement, the odds of having to seek medical aid greatly increase.)

- Eating a meal can trigger the gastrocolic reflex and thus cause a bowel movement approximately 30 to 60 minutes afterwards.

A few warning signs:

- The person has a prior history of rectal, anal, or other bowel problems. (You *did* check this before you started stuffing things up there, didn't you?)

- The person develops cramping abdominal pain, other bothersome abdominal pain, fever, or blood starts coming from their rectum. If any of these appear, it's time to see a physician immediately.
- The object hasn't passed on its own after 24 hours. Again, it's now time to see a doc.

What to Do When a Condom Fails

For men: OK, guy, while having intercourse you look down and see that the condom you were wearing has broken and you are now wearing a small latex ring around the base of your cock. Or maybe you look down and discover that the condom is gone. (You were thinking that this particular brand caused very little loss of sensation.) Perhaps you have already come. What do you do now?

STOP! Then, first of all, if she doesn't already know, you gotta tell her. Try not to sound too alarmed (she may regard what has happened as a big deal, or she may not), but let her know what happened.

OK, you told her. Now what? If you're worried about getting a sexually transmitted disease, go into the bathroom and wash your genitals several times with generous amounts of soap and water, then empty your bladder (and maybe drink fluids so you can flush out your urethra some more. One nurse who worked in an urban STD clinic told me that washing and urinating after sex would reduce a man's chances of getting gonorrhea by 50%. She had no statistics on whether it reduced his chances of getting some other diseases – but it's certain that washing and peeing can't hurt and could help quite a bit.)

For women: A woman is in a riskier situation. Trying to douche out your semen (and whatever it contains) may drive some of it further up into her body. Experts no longer recommend the use of nonoxynol-9 and other spermicides under such circumstances.

The first thing she can do is what I just recommended for men: wash her external genitals thoroughly with soap and water, and empty her bladder.

In addition, some new allies are available to help both of you through this situation. Different brands of "morning-after" pills can do a good job of preventing unwanted pregnancies. And new post-exposure protocols can help prevent you from catching a sexually transmitted disease, or keep it from affecting you as badly. Both types of treatments should ideally be started within 24 hours of exposure, or within 72 hours maximum – so seek help as soon as possible.

What to Do About a Latex Allergy

Latex allergies are becoming increasingly common - more and more hospitals have switched to non-latex products to protect their patients and staff. The nasty thing about this allergy is that it can appear quite suddenly, and dangerously, in someone who's never before had any trouble with latex.

Fortunately, there are good alternatives to latex for all your safer-sex needs. Polyurethane condoms are now available in both male and female versions, and have the added benefit of being impervious to oil-based lubricants. Gloves are available in nitrile and vinyl. While dental dams are always, as far as I know, made of latex, plastic wrap offers an inexpensive and effective alternative. So don't give up on safer sex - just switch products.

There are two types of latex allergy: contact dermatitis of the skin and systemic anaphylactic reaction.

A skin rash or itchiness after exposure to latex is usually nothing to worry about for now. Wash the affected area thoroughly to remove any traces of the latex, and use a standard over-the-counter anti-itch cream until the rash fades. However, it appears that such dermatitis can be an early sign of a more serious latex allergy on the way, so you should probably switch to non-latex products from now on, and talk to your doctor about a prescription for an Epi-Pen™ (more about those in a moment).

If you or your partner begins to have trouble breathing after exposure to latex, this is an emergency! This allergy can lead to swelling in the mouth and throat that renders the sufferer unable to breathe at all. (The reaction is the same type you've read about in the cases where someone dies after being stung by a bee.) If the breathing doesn't get noticeably easier almost right away, call 911 for an ambulance. Meanwhile, your first line of defense, if you have one, is the aforementioned Epi-Pen - a portable, easy-to-use, disposable syringe that delivers a jolt of a drug called epinephrine which will reduce the allergic reaction until you can get to the hospital for further treatment.

If you're allergic to latex, the allergy can impact your life outside the bedroom too (particularly in the area of health care). For more information, visit the website of the American Latex Allergy Association at *www.latexallergyresources.org* and check the "Help With Problems" section.

Male Sexual Emergencies

Men's sexual anatomies, being largely external to the rest of our bodies, are more prone than women's to various kinds of physical traumas – most of which are painful but minor, a few of which are serious. In addition, of course, there are general sexual emergencies that affect everybody. A highly readable and quite entertaining book on this topic is "Sex Disasters... And How to Survive Them," by Charles Moser., Ph.D., M.D., and Janet W. Hardy (Greenery Press, 2001); it covers most of this ground in detail, so I'm not going to spend a whole lot of time here. But below are a few of the more common sexual emergencies of which men should be aware:

Erections that won't: When she tells you that it happens to all men sooner or later, she's right. The best thing to do for now is don't sweat it. Figure out something you both enjoy that doesn't require an erection, and do that; then figure out something else, and do that; and so on, until you've both had a good enough time that you've forgotten about the erection for now. Odds on, it'll be back next time, when you're not so tired or distracted. If this turns into an ongoing problem, check out some literature on the problem, or talk to a doctor or sex therapist. Viagra and other, newer drugs can also be of tremendous assistance – there's an essay about Viagra later on in this book.

Genital trauma: Most men, by the time they reach adulthood, have had the experience of having their testicles hit, and know how excruciating it is. They also know that generally the pain is transitory – you don't really die, you just wish you had. Occasionally accidents happen during sex – someone gets clumsy climbing over someone else, or some such problem – and a knee goes somewhere that it shouldn't. Not much can be done except to apologize profusely and wait for the pain to die down, which it should do within an hour. Ice packs will help. If there's significant swelling, or if the pain doesn't go away within an hour, something may have gotten ruptured or twisted – get him to a doctor.

An unusual but not unheard-of injury is fracture of the penis, or "broken dick" – one of the balloon-like sacs that holds the blood inside the penis gets ruptured. This often happens during vigorous inter-course when the receptive partner is on top and the penis slips out of place and gets reinserted and "bent." You'll be able to tell this has happened because the penis will be very bruised and hanging crookedly, and it'll usually be quite painful. See a doctor promptly.

Priapism: A quite serious, male sexual emergency is "priapism" – an erection that lasts four hours or more. This condition happens sometimes in association with some prescription or street drugs, as well as some diseases such as sickle cell anemia. Priapism calls for an immediate emergency room visit.

Heart attack: No section on emergencies would be complete without a mention of the fact that men, particularly older men, often have heart attacks during sex. If you are the partner of a man over the age of 45 or so, it would be a very, very good idea for you to take a basic CPR class, and to maintain those skills – regardless of your sex life, the chances that you would be the person with him were he to have a heart attack are very good indeed, and you could be the person to save his life under those circumstances.

If you are having sex with anybody, and they complain of pain, fullness or uncomfortable pressure in their chest, shortness of breath, pain radiating down either arm or up into their jaw, or chest discomfort accompanied by nausea, sweating, pale skin, fainting or light-headedness, and the symptoms persist for more than ten minutes even with rest, stop doing whatever it is you're doing. Then call 911 – do not attempt to drive them to the hospital yourself.

building the perfect nightstand

Assuming most of your sexual activity takes place in your bed, it helps to keep the following supplies nearby, possibly in your nightstand.

• Something non-alcoholic to drink. This may help relieve the sometimes considerable thirst people can work up. If she's not wild about having someone come in her mouth, but willing to let him, keeping a strongly flavored liquid close by can help quickly wash the taste away.

• A music source that requires little attention. Auto-reverse and repeat features are useful. While tastes vary, many people prefer instrumental music. Lyrics can distract, and they're often about unpleasant topics.

• Soft, small towels kept nearby help with clean-up. (Many hookers refer to these as "trick towels.") If you leave a large wet spot, consider placing a very absorbent towel under you before things get serious.

• Lubricants make life easier. Make sure they're in containers that can be easily opened with slippery hands. If you use water-soluble lubricants, also keep a small "finger bowl" of water handy so you can add a few drops as necessary. (Don't add too much water. Doing so can wash most of the lube away.)

- Condoms, foams, suppositories, and other protective devices must be kept very close by. Remember, if you don't keep it handy, you won't take the time to use it.
- Incense can help create a wonderful atmosphere.
- Candles or a dimmable light source also help create a special, erotic atmosphere.
- A small flashlight can be useful in any number of situations. If you're experimenting with bondage, make sure you also have a "blackout light" (a light which plugs into a household outlet, and which automatically turns on in case of a power failure) in place.

A well-stocked nightstand contributes a lot toward helping your erotic play proceed smoothly. Rummaging through drawers, tramping off to the bathroom, or needing to make a quick trip to the kitchen can "break the spell" the two of you are creating. A small amount of planning ahead is well worth it.

Traveling Supplies

For several years now, I have made it a point to always carry a few condoms, a pair of latex gloves and some small (grape-sized) packs of lubricant in my jacket pocket. These inexpensive, readily portable supplies have enabled me to have several delightful (if somewhat unexpected) evenings that I otherwise would not have had. You never know when a wonderful opportunity may present itself. As the Boy Scouts say, "Be prepared."

items to avoid

While some items found in the ordinary household can be adapted in a safe and pleasurable way to improve sex, other items have such a high potential for causing emotional upsets or serious injury that I feel I must recommend against their use.

Please avoid using:

- Candles other than plain paraffin candles such as you find for emergency or Hanukkah use. As a rule, the harder the candle, the higher its melting point temperature, and thus the less suitable its wax is for dripping on skin. Colored or scented candles may also melt at a higher temperature than plain white candles. An exception may be the kind of candles sold in tall glasses, sometimes with religious paintings on the outside; these are sometimes made of extremely soft wax which melts at a very low temperature, often lower than the water you use to shower with. However, check all wax on your own body before dripping it on a partner, just to be sure.
- Clothes irons.
- Curling irons.
- Heavy-duty kitchen knives, hunting knives, and similar items with an extremely sharp cutting edge or point.
- Electric shock devices.
- Formal weapons such as firearms, swords, and tear-gas devices.

- Fireplace equipment.
- Hot rollers.
- Open flame other than a candle's flame.
- Sewing needles.
- Vacuum cleaners of any sort.

Some of the items listed above, particularly electric shock devices and knives, can be used during BDSM play by people who have first received expert instruction in their usage. (Not provided by this book.) People wanting to use such devices should contact a local BDSM club to receive adequate instruction prior to attempting to use those items.

Also, please avoid being sexual while operating a motor vehicle. I can understand that it may have its attractions, but it can distract the driver to a genuinely dangerous degree. I have a paramedic friend who has seen the all-too-grisly results that such distractions can produce.

how to clean toys after use

Attempting to sterilize a toy is usually neither necessary nor practical. You can, however, remove or kill so many microorganisms that there aren't enough to transmit a disease. (The saying that "it only takes one" is just simply not true. It often takes several million.) In other words, you can reduce their number below an "infectious concentration" and make it difficult or impossible for them to multiply.

Bugs are just like us in many ways. They need water, protection from extremes of heat and cold, something to eat, shielding from toxins, and a means of reproducing. If any of these gets disrupted too badly, soon the bugs won't exist any more.

Imagine that your favorite sex toy is lying over there on the ground with numerous nasty bugs on it. How might you clean it?

First of all, ask yourself a few questions. They'll determine what approach you take.

Who will this item be used on in the future? If it will only be used in the vagina or mouth of one person, decontamination isn't such a major issue. (If it's been in anybody's rectum and may eventually be in someone's vagina or mouth, or has been in the vagina of someone who has a yeast or other vaginal infection, cleaning is difficult, so use a condom on the toy to help prevent further contamination.)

Let's assume it's something you can get wet. First turn on some gently running warm water. Then put on latex (or other nonporous) gloves, pick up the item, and place it under the stream for a few minutes. Don't rush. What you're going for here is the physical removal of the bugs. Turn the item until all surfaces have been thoroughly exposed.

If the item is absorbent, such as a "jelly" or latex item, and you know that it's only going to be used on the person it was previously used on, you might stop here. Absorbent toys can retain various cleaning agents which can cause irritation or other problems later. Place the item on a low-lint cloth, or other place where it won't pick up any foreign bodies, and allow it to dry.

If the item is nonabsorbent, such as a plastic, silicone, or metal item, rinse it, scrub it with soap for a few minutes, then rinse again. (Simply placing the toy in the top rack of the dishwasher can be an excellent way to accomplish the entire cleaning process.) Don't underestimate the value of this step. A thorough washing with soap and water can remove up to 97% of all bugs.

Soap note: Certain types of soaps kill bugs better than others. In particular, nonscented, liquid soaps containing triclosan (generally labeled "antibacterial") are highly recommended.

Plug-in vibrators and battery-operated vibrators can be wiped with a cloth moistened with bleach solution or alcohol. If you use bleach, a "follow-up" wiping with water or alcohol will be needed to remove any bleach residue. Be sure not to get the "innards" wet.

If you believe that the item needs a more thorough decontamination, you can soak it in a number of cleaning solutions. Remember this principle: soak for *a minimum of 20 minutes.*

Nonabsorbent items can be washed, then soaked in a solution made from nine parts water to one part 5.25% sodium hypochlorite bleach (common household bleach) for at least 20 minutes. This is a very powerful disinfectant with a very broad spectrum. It is the preferred cleaning agent. Be sure to use a bleach-water solution that's not more than a few hours old. Rinse with water or alcohol to remove any bleach residue. After rinsing, set the item aside to dry.

Nonabsorbent, and some absorbent, items can be soaked for at least 20 minutes in a solution containing at least 60% ethanol or isopropyl alcohol. Alcohol evaporates rapidly, so it may be wise to use a covered container. Note that alcohol is not as broad spectrum a decontaminant as bleach and water.

Metal objects can be brought to a brief boil and then allowed to cool. Note: New studies show that once water has been brought to a boil, everything that can be killed by boiling has been killed, and thus more prolonged boiling is unnecessary.

Leather items such as whips can be very difficult to clean. Wipe them down with soapy water, then wipe them again with alcohol (bleach is more likely to decolorize the leather), and set them aside to dry. They may need to be reconditioned afterwards.

Allowing an item to dry is a frequently under-appreciated means of decontamination. Many microorganisms need a moist environment to survive, and either die or become incapable of causing infection after a few hours in a dry environment. Simply allowing an item to dry for several hours, or better yet several days, will result in substantial decontamination. This process can be enhanced if coupled with even a few minutes of exposure to direct sunlight.

A quiet note about handwashing: more frequent handwashing can do a lot to decrease the spread of infectious disease. (It dramatically reduces the spread of the common cold, for example.) The protective value of washing your hands after you play, and after you clean your toys, is not yet fully appreciated.

Cleaning toys can seem like something of a chore at first, but with time it becomes "just another part of it." Also, the time spent cleaning your toys can be a delicious time to contemplate how, when, and on whom they'll next be used.

Viagra® – what's really going on?

- *What is Viagra?* Viagra is the commercial name for a drug called sildenafil citrate.
- *How does it work?* Viagra increases the amount of blood that flows into the penis and increases how long it stays there. This allows a man to have a firmer erection for a longer period of time.
- *Is it an aphrodisiac?* No. While Viagra makes it easier for a man to get an erection, and to keep it once he gets it, it does not cause sexual arousal or an increase in libido.
- *What does Viagra do for women?* Some recent studies have shown that Viagra can sometimes help women who are experiencing a decrease in libido due to taking other medications. See your doctor for more information.
- *How long does it last?* Viagra reaches an effective level in the bloodstream about 30 to 60 minutes after it has been taken, and its effects last for at least four hours.
- *Who should take it?* Assuming its use is otherwise appropriate, Viagra should be taken by men who have trouble maintaining an adequate erection. Nearly half of all men over the age of 40 have this problem to at least some degree. This is sometimes due to a serious underlying physical condition such as diabetes or high blood pressure so it is important to be examined by a doctor before starting to use it.

- *What are the major risks?* The major risk involves mixing Viagra with nitrate-type drugs that lower blood pressure, such as nitroglycerin tablets. Doing so can cause the blood pressure to drop to a dangerously low level.

- *What are the alternatives?* Some natural herbs and some alternative prescription medications are available, as well as some mechanical treatments. For more information on those, consult the websites below or ask your physician.

- *If a man takes Viagra, will his penis stay erect after he has had an orgasm?* The man will likely have a normal decrease in penis size after orgasm, however he may find it easier to later have a second erection.

- *Does using Viagra cause heart attacks?* No. However, men with certain heart conditions should limit their sexual activity as advised by their physicians, whether or not they use Viagra.

For more information:

www.viagra.com

www.treatments-for-erectile-dysfunction.com

www.webmd.com

- *Are there other drugs that do the same thing as Viagra?* Yes, and more seem to be on the way. The best-known of the "new Viagras" is a drug called Levitra – you can learn more about it at *www.levitra.com*. A lot of research is taking place in this area, and it seems certain that more new drugs will be appearing in the next few years, so keep in touch with your doctor to learn more.

sex and the law

Sexual behavior is subject to numerous laws. All countries have laws that regulate sexual conduct. In the United States, there are both federal and state laws that regulate sexual conduct. While a lot of people have a sort of "common law" understanding of what those laws are, very few have actually looked up the relevant statutes. Note: While I've researched and studied this area, I am not a lawyer and the following should not be regarded as legal advice.

At both the state and federal level, there are three general categories of "laws" in the United States. All three branches of government, including the legislative branch, the executive branch, and the judicial branch "make law" in various ways. The legislature makes law by passing statutes. The executive branch makes law by putting out various regulations – such as those from OSHA and the FCC, for example. The judicial branch makes law by applying the statutes passed by the legislature to the facts of the cases that come before it. (Note: this often has a huge effect on the meaning of a law and how it will or won't be enforced, and is one of the main issues in legal research.) When I use the term "law" in this article I am generally referring to statutes passed by a state legislature or by Congress.

Note regarding executive regulations: the penalties for violating a regulation put out by an executive branch typically do not involve jail time and thus are subject to more informal "administrative hearings" instead of actual trials. However their rulings can usually be appealed to the regular court system.

Note regarding judicial authority: there are generally three levels of courts at both the state and federal level – trial courts, appellate courts, and supreme courts. In a given jurisdiction, whether state or federal, usually several trial courts are under the "umbrella" of a particular appellate court and all of the appellate courts are under the umbrella of the supreme court. The higher the court's authority, the more binding are its rulings on the courts below it. Rulings by a state's supreme court are binding on all future similar cases that come before the courts in that particular state, and rulings by the United States Supreme Court are binding on all courts in the country.

The relevant federal laws are found in what's called the United States Code. This code is organized into what are called titles. Each title is divided into parts. The parts are divided into chapters and each chapter is divided into sections. The sections contain the actual wording of the particular offense. For example, the federal law regarding what is called "aggravated sexual abuse" is found in Title 19, Part I, Chapter 109A, Section 2241 of the United States Code. Many states model their laws closely on federal laws, so looking over the federal laws can give you a good general idea of what you're likely to find as you look over a state's codes. Note also that there is a federal requirement that such laws be written in "plain English" so they are likely to be much easier to read than a state's laws are.

Regarding studying the laws around sexual behavior (and virtually everything else), we currently live in an era of "I've got some good news and I've got some bad news."

The good news is that it's now pretty easy to look up the wording of the actual statutes. In the old days, a person seeking such knowledge often had to go to a public library to look over the basic books containing the statutes. (Many, if not most, public libraries still have such books; they're usually found in the library's reference section.) If the person wanted to also look over the cases that interpreted these laws, they often had to go to a law library – and that can be a very daunting place unless you've had prior training in how to find your way around. Nowadays, the situation is better. All state laws, and all federal laws, and many of the cases that interpret these laws, can be found online. The laws and cases of many other countries can also be found online.

The bad news is that carefully looking over the various statutes may not give you the full picture. Reading the statutes, regulations, and cases, will give you a fairly good overall picture, but there's more. Law enforcement officers, prosecutors, and judges often have what's called "discretion" in how aggressively they will enforce a particular law. What that means is that different jurisdictions place a higher or lower priority on how much of their limited time and other resources they will devote to a particular violation of the law. For example, arrest and prosecution for possession of a small amount of marijuana may be a very low priority, but arrest and prosecution for domestic violence may be a high priority.

While you could call your local district attorney's office and ask them what the "hot items of the day" are, if you're really curious about a particular issue it just might be a whole lot smarter to contact a private attorney, or maybe the public defenders office – they may be too busy to do much to help you unless you've actually been arrested – and have them make inquiries on your behalf. (Your attorney will keep your name confidential unless you're stupid enough to say something like, "I'm gonna kill my wife tomorrow!")

Here are some legal questions you might see if you can research and get an answer to:

1. Exactly how "affectionate" can I become with my partner before we put ourselves at risk for being arrested for public indecency?

2. I left my X-rated videos in an unlocked box while I was at work and my teen-age son was at home alone. Am I at risk of being charged with something like "contributing to the delinquency of a minor"?

3. Is it against the law in my state for me to have anal sex with my boyfriend?

4. What is the age of consent in my state? Is it different for girls and boys? Does any difference in our age matter?

5. Is bestiality a crime in my state? How is it defined?

6. What acts constitute rape in my state?

7. I've heard that my neighbors have "wife swapping" parties. Are those legal?

8. A woman I've been having sex with is pregnant and claims that the child is mine. She is going to keep the baby. Will I have to pay child support for the next 18 years?

9. If someone who has AIDS or herpes has sex with me and doesn't tell me first and I get infected, can I sue them? Can they be arrested?

10. How is prostitution defined in my state? If my wife insists upon working in a house of prostitution over my objections, can I be arrested for pimping?

11. Does having sex with my second cousin constitute incest?

12. I married my wife when she was 16 years old and I carry around a wedding night picture of her sucking my cock. Am I guilty of possessing child pornography?

Here are some useful URLs that you can use to assist you in your research.

www.law.cornell.edu – this is a major legal portal to legal information of all kinds. It has an excellent section on federal laws. Actually, all of its sections are excellent.

www.catalaw.com – a good resource for legal information regarding the United States and other countries. Choose "sexuality law" from their list of topics.

www.lectlaw.com/tsex.htm – the 'Lectric Law Library is a genuine treasure. Interesting, funny, and well organized. Good section on sexuality law. Good sections on many, many other things.

www.yahoo.com – relevant area is the website directory towards the bottom of the main page. Choose "society and culture" then either "legal issues" or "sex crimes" and go from there.

www.nolo.com – an excellent legal resource. Hard to beat it as a "start here" spot for learning about any legal topic. Only major negative is not many links to outside sources.

www.freeadvice.com – excellent free website offering a wide range of legal information.

www.ageofconsent.com – a good listing of age of consent laws for the United States and other countries.

www.sexlaws.org – a very good and informative website. Emphasis in on the laws concerning sexual assault and statutory rape. Good useful links. You can also get to the main page of this site by going to *www.statutoryrape.org* and www.sexualassault.org.

www.lawforkids.org – this website, funded by the Arizona Supreme Court, is an excellent legal education site for just about any legal topic, including those related to sex. While the emphasis is, of course, on Arizona law, it's an excellent site for general legal education.

some resources for further exploring your sexuality

I've chosen a "gateway" resource for each of these forms of alternative sexuality. Visiting most any of these websites will lead you to dozens of other helpful resources.

General Questions about Alternative Sexuality
Society for Human Sexuality, *www.sexuality.org*
San Francisco Sex Information, *www.sfsi.org*

Bisexuality
Bisexual Foundation, *www.bisexual.org*

Body Size
National Association to Aid Fat Acceptance, *www.naafa.org*

Corsetry
Corset College, *groups.yahoo.com/group/corsetcollege*

Crossdressing
Society for the Second Self, *www.tri-ess.org*

Expanded Families/Polyamory
Alt.polyamory homepage, *www.polyamory.org*

Gay/Lesbian
Gay Insider, *www.gayinsider.com*

Infantilism
Diaper Pail Fraternity, *www.dpf.com*

Piercing and Other Body Modifications
Body Play Magazine, *www.bodyplay.com/bodyplay*

Pleasure Parties
Passion Parties, *www.passionparties.com*

Sex Work
Bay Area Sex Worker Advisory Network, *www.bayswan.org*

Swinging
The Lifestyles Organization, *www.lifestyles.org*

SM
Society of Janus, *www.soj.org*

Tantra and Related Practices
The Resource for Tantra, Tantric Sex & The Kama Sutra, *www.tantra.com*

some resources for help with problems

Probably the most important advice I can give you regarding finding help for the problems listed below, and for other problems, is to grab your phone book and start looking. Many communities have local resources. Check the first few pages and look over the table of contents. Look up these and related topics in both the white and yellow pages. Check your phone book for an index.

Local newspapers and magazines, particularly free or low-cost ones that come out on a weekly or less frequent basis, often carry valuable listings. Gay and lesbian papers can be particularly helpful. Look them over carefully.

The Internet can be an excellent source of information for problems related to human sexuality; however, understand that the quality of information can vary widely. Thus the Latin saying *caveat literati* – "let the reader beware" – definitely applies here. Still, typing in certain phrases into a few different search engines can yield uncounted pages of information.

Gateway Resources

There are certain online "gateway resources" that lead to numerous other resources. They are:

San Francisco Sex Information, *www.sfsi.org*

Society for Human Sexuality, *www.sexuality.org*

Abuse/Battering/Neglect

National Domestic Violence Hotline
800 799-7233 *www.ndvh.org*

National Child Abuse Hotline
800 422-4453 *www.childehelpusa.org*

Parents Anonymous, *www.parentsanonymous.org*

AIDS

National AIDS Hotline, 800 342-AIDS *www.ashastd.org/nah,
www.aids.org*

Birth Control

Planned Parenthood, *www.plannedparenthood.org*

Censorship

American Civil Liberties Union, *www.aclu.org*

Electronic Frontier Foundation, *www.eff.org*

Circumcision

National Organization of Circumcision Information Resource Centers, *www.nocirc.org*

Disabilities

www.*disabledsex.org*

Herpes

www.herpes.org

Impotence

American Foundation for Urologic Disease, *www.impotence.org*

Incest

Survivors of Incest Anonymous, *www.siawso.org*

Latex Allergy

American Latex Allergy Association *www.latexallergyresources.org*

latexallergylinks.tripod.com

Use of the Epipen, *www.epipen.com*

Rape

Note: I was astonished to discover, in researching this book, a 2002 study from the Department of Justice that showed that one rape victim in eight is male.

National Organization Against Male Sexual Victimization, *www.malesurvivor.org*

People Against Rape *www.people-against-rape.org*

Stop Prison Rape *www.spr.org*

Sex Therapy

Sex Therapy Online, *www.sexology.org*

Sex and Love Addiction

Sexual Addiction Recovery Resources, *www.sarr.org*

Sexaholics Anonymous, *www.sa.org*

Stalking

Survivors of Stalking, *www.soshelp.org*

Suicidal/Homicidal Feelings

American Association of Suicidology
800 SUICIDE *www.suicidology.org*

Yellow Ribbon Suicide Prevention Programs (teen suicide), *www.yellowribbon.org*

some selected further readings

In addition to the books listed below, my publisher, Greenery Press, publishes many interesting books about both conventional and alternative sexualities. See the last page of this book for a complete listing.

Anal Pleasure and Health: A Guide for Men and Women by Jack Morin, Down There Press

The Good Vibrations Guide To Sex by Cathy Winks and Anne Semans, Cleis Press

Guide To Getting It On by Paul Joannides, Goofy Foot Press

How To Be A Great Lover by Lou Paget, Broadway Books

The Ultimate Guide to Anal Sex For Men by Bill Brent, Cleis Press

The Ultimate Guide To Fellatio by Violet Blue, Cleis Press

The New Joy Of Sex by Alex Comfort, Pocket Books

Sex Tips for Straight Women from a Gay Man by Dan Anderson, Regan Books

Trust, the Hand Book: A Guide to the Sensual and Spiritual Art of Handballing by Bert Herrman, Alamo Square Press

You Want Me To Do What? An Illustrated Book On The Joys Of Fellatio by Taylor

The Multi-Orgasmic Man: Sexual Secrets Every Man Should Know by Mantak Chia and Douglas Abrams

GENERAL SEXUALITY

Big Big Love: A Sourcebook on Sex for People of Size and Those Who Love Them
Hanne Blank
$15.95

The Bride Wore Black Leather... And He Looked Fabulous!: An Etiquette Guide for the Rest of Us
Andrew Campbell
$11.95

Erotic Tickling
Michael Moran
$12.95

The Ethical Slut: A Guide to Infinite Sexual Possibilities
Dossie Easton & Catherine A. Liszt
$16.95

A Hand in the Bush: The Fine Art of Vaginal Fisting
Deborah Addington
$13.95

Health Care Without Shame: A Handbook for the Sexually Diverse and Their Caregivers
Charles Moser, Ph.D., M.D.
$11.95

The Lazy Crossdresser
Charles Anders
$13.95

Look Into My Eyes: How to Use Hypnosis to Bring Out the Best in Your Sex Life
Peter Masters
$16.95

Phone Sex: Oral Thrills and Aural Skills
Miranda Austin
$15.95

Sex Disasters... And How to Survive Them
C. Moser, Ph.D., M.D. and Janet W. Hardy
$16.95

Tricks... To Please a Woman
by Jay Wiseman
$14.95

Turning Pro: A Guide to Sex Work for the Ambitious and the Intrigued
Magdalene Meretrix
$16.95

When Someone You Love Is Kinky
Dossie Easton & Catherine A. Liszt
$15.95

BDSM/KINK

The Bullwhip Book
Andrew Conway
$11.95

The Compleat Spanker
Lady Green
$12.95

Family Jewels: A Guide to Male Genital Play and Torment
Hardy Haberman
$12.95

Flogging
Joseph W. Bean
$11.95

Intimate Invasions: The Erotic Ins and Outs of Enema Play
M.R. Strict
$13.95

Jay Wiseman's Erotic Bondage Handbook
Jay Wiseman
$16.95

The Loving Dominant
John Warren
$16.95

Miss Abernathy's Concise Slave Training Manual
Christina Abernathy
$12.95

The Mistress Manual: The Good Girl's Guide to Female Dominance
Mistress Lorelei
$16.95

The New Bottoming Book
The New Topping Book
both by Dossie Easton & Janet W. Hardy
$14.95

The Seductive Art of Japanese Bondage
Midori
$27.95

The Sexually Dominant Woman: A Workbook for Nervous Beginners
Lady Green
$11.95

SM 101: A Realistic Introduction
Jay Wiseman
$24.95

Training With Miss Abernathy: A Workbook for Erotic Slaves and Their Owners
Christina Abernathy
$13.95

FICTION

.. But I Know What You Want: 25 Sex Tales for the Different
James Williams
$13.95

Haughty Spirit
Sharon Green
$11.95

Love, Sal: letters from a boy in The City
Sal Iacopelli, ill. Phil Foglio
$13.95

Murder At Roissy
John Warren
$15.95

The Warrior Within
The Warrior Enchained
both by Sharon Green
$11.95

Please include $3 for first book and $1 for each additional book with your order to cover shipping and handling costs, plus $10 for overseas orders. VISA/MC accepted. Order from Greenery Press, 3403 Piedmont Ave. #301, Oakland, CA 94611, 510/652-2596, www.greenerypress.com